1

To Léontine

THE ANTI-AGING DIET:
REVERSE
THE BIOLOGICAL
CLOCK !

Alain ANDREU

Translated from French by Olivia Scott

"The cradle rocks above an abyss, and common
sense tells us that our existence is but a brief crack
of light between two eternities of darkness."
Vladimir Nabokov, *Speak, Memory*.

DISCLAIMER

This work is the result of a personal journey, the aim of which is to improve ones health and to reduce the effects of time. Despite working in the medicinal field for 30 years, this author is not a doctor, and advises to consult a doctor before making the decision to take any food supplement or hormonal therapy. In fact, in this book you will find information on health that is off the beaten track from "conventional medicine". The anti-age protocol of functional and nutritional medicine that you will discover is preventative medicine. Even if you're not sick, it's about optimizing your health and preventing disease. It's a small price to pay for a long and healthy life.

ABOUT THE AUTHOR

For nearly thirty years I have worked in a biology and medical laboratory, as part of an institute of research situated in the middle of the Pacific, in French Polynesia.

From the age of about forty years old, I started to suffered from perverse effects linked to aging and the imbalance of hormones that comes with it: chronic back pain, metabolic syndrome, gastroesophageal reflux, weight gain, fatigue. Plus, I hadn't participated in any sort of sports activity since my thirties.

Furthermore, early health problems (two melanomas at age thirty, Hashimoto's thyroiditis at the same age, a repeat of basal cell carcinoma and Scheuermann's disease which caused my spine to grow) had demotivated me a little when it came to physical activities outdoors, living in a tropical country and in addition to being a red phenotype (fair-skinned).

Like many of us, I was fatalistic and I thought that after all, if the doctors and physiotherapists I consulted regularly could not solve my problem; I certainly could not do it myself. I thought (wrongly) that it was useless to fight against unfavorable genetics and that I should resign myself to accepting things how they were. However, this fragile health impacted my professional life more and more. The lack of energy affected both my mental and physical abilities to the point that I realized it was urgent to do something if I wanted to stay in the race.

Where do you start then, when after a career in a medical field, you suddenly realize conventional medicine is unable to cure most chronic diseases (type 2 diabetes, osteoarthritis) To tell the truth, I had never addressed this question on health before: how to improve it by means other than chemical, by using other ways than those which are fed to us by big laboratories and the health system. Until then, my only reflections were rather philosophical. At that time I regularly wrote critical analysis's of the work of Vladimir Nabokov for the American magazine *The Nabokovian* (hence the quote on the cover page!) and I did not care much about the content of my plate.

So, I had to open up my mind to alternative medicine, sort through the contradictory information that filled the internet about nutrition and official nutritional recommendations from PNNS (The French National Nutrition and Health Program), dissect through scientific publications. The latest health scandals that shook the Afssaps ((French Agency for Health Product Safety) who later became ANSM after the Mediator affair) in recent years, as well as those in progress or to come (statins, Depakine®, Levothyrox® etc.) added to my growing skepticism about conventional medicine.

- "Good, good." said my editor, with a satisfied air, closing the manuscript with a heavy hand. But why write an expensive book about it?

I wrote this book because I see people suffering unnecessarily from the effects of aging every day. This book is primarily intended for these people, to help them gain control of their health, and benefit from my own experience. The body is a complex machinery that requires a holistic approach: environment, stress, nutrition, hormones and micronutrients. They are all intimately connected and there is no such thing as a miracle pill. If you are amongst those who still think that osteoarthritis is treated with anti-inflammatories, osteoporosis with bisphosphonates, atherosclerosis with statins, then I'm afraid you spent money for nothing and I invite you to stop wasting your time and offer this book to a friend instead!

If, on the other hand, you are ready to try the adventure of anti-aging medicine (anti-aging or reverse aging medicine) by agreeing to change your daily life, you will soon start to feel the following effects: weight loss, new-found energy, positive mentality, a metamorphosed body, less pain.

Ua reva, as they say in French Polynesia, here we go!

PART 1

WHY THIS BOOK IS MADE FOR YOU

Because you are the star of your own health and you can take control of it.

In fact, if you apply the basic rules of this book, you will quickly realize the impact that that can have on your body and mentality beyond your belief.

Because the patient is always right !

It was the grandfather of doctor Thierry Hertoghe, Eugène Hertoghe, one of the pioneers of hypothyroid hormone therapy, who always said that. Unfortunately, a thorough clinical exam can obviously not be done in ten minutes of consultation. More than often, the doctor does not listen to the patient's complaints or take them seriously enough. It is for that reason that I advise you to play an active role in the improvement of your own health. This book does not promote self-medication, its aim, rather, is to encourage the reader to take charge in a preventative way.

Indeed, "official" medicine waits for you to fall ill in order to treat you. It it is an emergency medicine, usually very effective, which saves lives. For example, look at the progress that has been made on infections since the discovery of penicillin. For chronic illnesses, however, the results aren't so pretty and the majority of proposed treatments are symptomatic and do not solve the problem. This comes from the fact that medicine considers the patient as a set of organs, often treated separately, while chronic illnesses require a holistic (global) approach to be overcome.

Anti-aging medicine is part of this approach: it is necessary to optimize your health, in order to prevent falling ill. Because, whatever anyone says, to grow old is to accept a decrease in health. Why then, should we support unnecessary suffering if we can avoid it by living better and for longer? You will see that a lot of illnesses considered as being an unstoppable part of aging like arthritis, type II diabetes, hypertension, cancer and even androgenic alopecia can be overcome or prevented with a global approach.

WHAT IS AGING?

Many phenomenons interact with and make the body more vulnerable as it gets older: glycation, oxidation, chronic inflammation, telomere shortening and hormonal failure. According to certain authors, immunity equally plays an important part in life expectancy.

Let's look at this in further detail.

GLYCATION

Glycation is a chemical reaction that take place between a sugar and a protein, giving a sort of non-functional aggregate which, once oxidized in the organism, becomes what we call an A.G.E (Advanced Glycation End-product).

These products of advanced/progressive glycation or AGE, harm the kidneys, the heart and eyes. It's the "Maillard" reaction: one could say that our body "caramelizes" and that our arteries lose their elasticity with this phenomenon. The opacification of crystallin, or cataract, is a direct consequence of these AGEs.

Our bodies produce them every day but more still with industrial foods and junk food such as: sugary breakfast cereals, meat cooked at high temperatures (barbecue), fries and sodas.

Even hemoglobin, the protein which is found in our red blood cells, suffers the effects of sugar by partially transforming it into glycated hemoglobin or HbA1c. This glycated hemoglobin remains in the red blood cell during the entire cell life cycle which is around 120 days. That's why it's used for to monitor diabetes in the laboratory because it gives the practitioner a clear idea of sugar consumption in recent weeks while fasting plasma glucose is only a "snippet" at the given time of the blood test.

As you will have understood: sugar accelerates the aging process, the studies prove it (1).

The damages of glycation being both important and irreversible, the anti-aging medicine strongly insists on prevention as it will be more effective along with nutritional advice. There is also a supplement, carnosine (which is naturally found in meat, hence the name), is capable of reducing the production of AGE's. It is linked to an improvement of life expectancy in the animal (2).

OXIDATIVE STRESS

Evidence was found for **oxidative stress** in 1956 by Dr. Denham Harman and its role in aging has now been universally accepted. Simply breathing, and therefore being in contact with oxygen, produces free radicals. A polluted environment, physical activity and overeating all generate oxidation and damage our bodies. Fortunately, this one generates a certain number of molecules, enzymes (superoxide dismutase among other), glutathione, coenzyme Q10, lipoid acid and melatonin are all antioxidants that our body is lead to produce each day. Glutathione, to name just one example, is often found in low quantities in patients who suffer from Parkinson's disease, and its administration slows the formation of the disease.

Glutathione is quite unstable in the body's exterior but there is an inexpensive nutritional precursor supplement of gluthatione called N-Acetyl-Cystein (NAC) (3).

So, is it sufficient enough to supplement oneself with antioxidants in order to protect against the effects of aging? Unfortunately, recent studies show that oxidative stress seems necessary in order to make the body protect itself and that an over-consummation of antioxidant supplements would be harmful, except for patients suffering from degenerative illnesses (Parkinson's, AMD). This is how the oxidative stress produced by sport is beneficial for health because it forces the body to adapt (4).

To find out more about ones own anti-radical status, there are urinary and blood tests that test for oxidative stress which have been around for some time now. In the UK, one can find oxidative stress tests here: https://smartnutrition.co.uk/health-tests/oxidative-stress/. Be that as it may, the rule of caution with regards to supplementation is to always stay within the recommended physiological dose so that your body can absorb it or doesn't over-produce. This also applies to bio-identical hormones, as we will see later.

INFLAMMATION

Chronic inflammation is still an under-estimated phenomenon, and which is usually only treated once it gets to a critical level with the help of a well-known marker such as CRP (or c-reactive protein) or possibly fibrinogen. However, these classic markers do not detect low levels of inflammation despite being responsible for most cardiovascular diseases. We now know that cholesterol is not to blame for atheroscleroses, and that the formation of atheroma plaque is probably provoked by inflammation of the artery lining. We could accuse calcium as much as cholesterol which has been found in equal amounts in atheroma plaque but it's a long story and the sugar industry in particular has decided otherwise. (5,6 and7)

That is how the **high-sensitivity CRP** test was created: to be able to measure with precision the rate of lower CRP to 5mg/l and give an idea of the level of chronic inflammation. This test is now, with **homocysteine**, known as one of the best indicators of cardiovascular risk, much better than the classic lipid abnormality test, which has been prescribed for decades.

Regular intake of A.I.N.S (non-steroidal anti-inflammatory drugs) has been shown to significantly reduce the risk of colon, breast, prostate and esophageal cancer. For Alzheimer's disease, the risk would be lowered by 75%!

There are some who take a daily administration of 100mg of aspirin to limit inflammation, especially in the USA, but it is actually quite easy to reduce the level of inflammation with a suitable diet. This includes an intake of EDA/DHA fatty acids (omega 3, found in oily fish or rapeseed oil), taking certain spices (turmeric, clove, ginger) or certain plants that have amazing anti-TNF-alpha properties (see chapter on alopecia).

TELOMERE SHORTENING

Telomeres are the outer pieces of ADN forming our chromosomes. Their discovery, along with the enzyme telomerase, which takes care of their integrity, was made the object of a Nobel prize in 2009.

In each division, the cell loses a bit of its telomeres, and finishes by dying. It is one of the explanations of aging. Telomerase activators such as **epitalon** (protein peptide) and **astragalus** derivatives (TA65) are new anti-aging tools used by physicians in functional medicine albeit slightly expensive. These telomerase activators contain cycloastragenol, an active principle held in very small quantities in the Astragale plan, and of which the extraction process is costly. Equally, there are laboratory tests that allow us to measure the length of our telomeres as well as knowing our biological age. But these tests need to be a little more standardized - the difference notably seems to have been written by those which tested them (8).

HORMONE DEFICIENCY

Finally, the **hormone rate**, in general optimizes around 25 years, decreasing regularly with age in particular with the following hormones: DHEA, growth hormone, sexual hormones, melatonin, and even thyroidal hormones. It is for this reason that it is advised to always establish a hormonal checkup around the age of 25. This is in order to use it as a basis for hormonal therapy that we will use later.

These deficiencies come more or less quickly, according to the genetics of the individual, and of course their way of living. This is how we know who amongst us are younger than their marital status: it is what we call

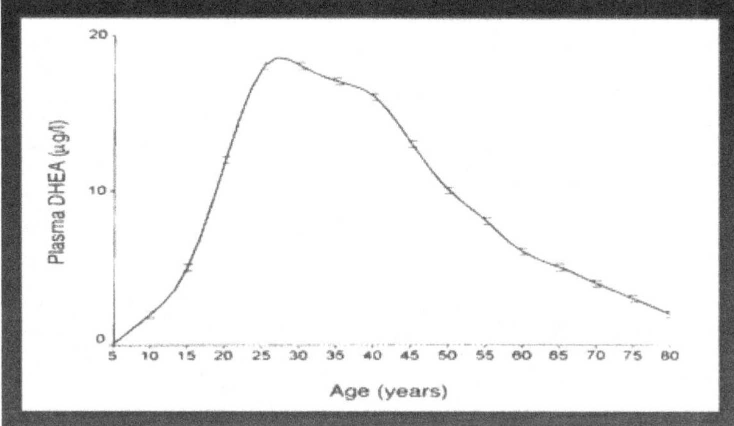

the biological age. Anti-aging physicians have a range of tests to assess the biological age of their patients, and hormonal testing is one of them.

THE PROBLEM OF LABORATORY STANDARDS

FREQUENT VALUES

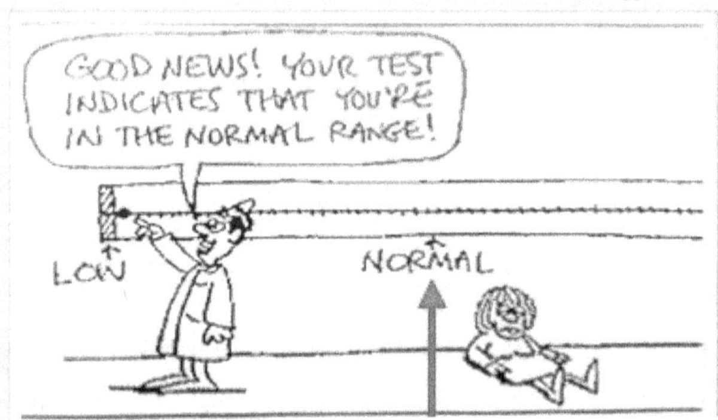

In theory, each laboratory should establish its "standards" or "frequency means" according to its recruitment in order to respond to a given population. In practice, the values given to the patient are quite often those supplied by the manufacturers reagent kit.

These values are established according to the following assumption: it is estimated that only 5% of the population - that being 2 people out of 40 - are situated outside the norm. In other words, these values assume that

95% of the population are in a normal biological situation.

If we compare things with sight problems, it would be to treat those who are partially blind and leave behind the majority of myopes, astigmatisms and other presbytes whose sight deserves a small correction!

That is how a lot of us have experienced their doctor telling them "everything will be fine!" when reading a thyroid checkup with a TSH at 3mlU/L - not controlled by a thorough clinical examination and ignore our complaints of fatigue.

As you can see, the frequent laboratory values are in no way "health" values : do not let anyone convince you otherwise.

Even by "tightening" the interval to "optimize" the standards, as anti-aging medicine does, one must not lose sight of the fact that these values, for a given hormone, are to be compared with a clinical examination and the size of the patient. A tall man, for example, will need a greater level of testosterone and heightened IGF 1 than a man that is of average height or small.

HOW TO FIGHT AGAINST THE EFFECTS OF AGE?

This question seems to bother people, and it is not uncommon to hear that old age is a normal process of life, that would be futile to fight against. Yet, many studies highlight the conditions that accelerate - or slow - aging. According to some authors it could even be reversed to a certain extent. Anti-aging medicine, recently renamed "pro-aging medicine", does not really aim to extend the life span (even if it does) but rather to improve the quality of life that one calls DFLE, otherwise known as disability-free life expectancy. Contrary to popular belief, DFLE has been declining for several years. More worryingly, the last two years have seen a significant decline in life expectancy in all developed countries (9).

To summarize in geriatric terms, in recent years there has been an "increase in morbidity" and recently a reduction in unexplained life expectancy, not to mention the epidemic of obesity in most developed countries. This is what Dr. Thierry Hertoghe refers to as a "wheelchair prescription", and it is the choice of our current society, with its cortege of palliative care that makes the pharmaceutical industry happy.

However, there is a way to take care of biological aging in order to increase prolong the amount of healthy years thanks to the scientific advancement in hormonal and nutritional therapy of anti-aging medicine. Although all the anti-aging doctors will find you an abundance of studies to confirm the validity of their discipline, the best way to convince you of it is to test these treatment on oneself. Therefore, it was my curiosity and skeptical nature that lead me to do so.

The result has exceeded my expectations, hence the decision to write this ebook. Firstly to benefit the greatest number of people by sparing them years of research, and then for my friends, who frequently ask me for advice but unfortunately, I cannot explain everything in five minutes.

I'm sure that everyone will agree with me that spending the last years of their life in a nappy, taking stress medication, cholesterol, osteoarthritis, laser sessions for cataract or taking dietary supplements compared to adjusting their hormonal status, following a Paleolithic diet and doing sports three times a week; the second option is by far the most rewarding in terms of quality of life if we give ourselves the necessary means.

For indeed - I am going to let you in on a secret here - to have a good figure, a muscular, energetic body and an alert mind requires a multi-factorial approach that no pill, injection or ten-minute consultation with a GP can bring you. You have to attack the problem from all sides (we will see later that it is good to have a dietetic break from time to time. The weekend, for example, to preserve ones social life and give yourself time to "refuel"). This is the assumption of anti-aging medicine: activate the metabolism through nutrition, supplements, sports and adjust its hormonal status with identical organic hormones.

An encouraging movement was initiated in France with publishing houses specializing in advanced nutrition such as Thierry Souccar Editions, and his website www.lanutrition.fr. Jean Marc Dupuis and his letter from Santé Nature Innovation, expanded by a team of doctors

(Dr. Hertoghe, Dr. Rueff and others) have allowed the greatest number of people to access information on advanced remedies in alternative medicine.

Anti-aging medicine still has a reputation of being reserved for the wealthy and celebrities who can afford growth hormone injections, take telomerase activators, or receive stem cell treatment. We will see that this view is reductive. Having tested a good part of these treatments, I will explain further how to achieve good results at low cost.

Part 2

ARE FOOD SUPPLEMENTS DANGEROUS ?

Who has not already heard this statement from their doctor. Of course, this does not concern those prescribed by himself, available in pharmacies, and which are far from being irreproachable, as we will see.

The reality, which no one can dispute, is that drugs are responsible for around 20,000 deaths per year (10). As Professors Even and Debré teach, most medications are drugs that only relieve the symptoms rather than treating the cause. These authors estimate that nearly 40% of specialized drugs have little or no efficacy, 22% of these have been scientifically proven to have no effect whatsoever. Besides that, the accidents attributable to taking food supplements around the world are insignificant.

The goal of holistic medicine such as anti-aging medicine is precisely to prevent and limit the use of chemical molecules as much as possible, mostly non bio-identical, and a sometimes questionable risk assessment.

The common argument is that a good and varied diet is enough to cover all the daily needs of vitamins, fatty acids and minerals. This view is both wrong and obsolete. There is indeed an abundance of studies against this assertion. Below is a study by the company Geigy, who focus on a sharp decline in the nutritional value of food over the years.

Minerals in mg and vitamins by 100g		1985	1996	1996 compared with 1985	2002	2002 compared with 1985
Broccoli	Calcium	103	33	-68%	28	-73%
	Folic acid	47	23	-51%	18	-62%
	Magnesium	26	22	-15%	11	-58%
Beans	Calcium	56	34	-39%	22	-61%
	Folic acid	39	34	-13%	30	-23%
	Magnesium	26	22	-15%	18	-31%
Potatoes	Calcium	14	4	-71%	3	-79%
	Magnesium	27	18	-33%	14	-48%
Carrots	Calcium	37	31	-16%	28	-24%
	Magnesium	21	9	-57%	6	-71%
Spinach	Calcium	62	19	-69%	15	-76%
	Vitamin C	51	21	-59%	18	-65%
Apples	Vitamin C	5	1	-80%	2	-60%
Bananas	Calcium	8	7	-13%	7	-13%

	Folic acid	23	3	-87%	5	-78%
	Magnesium	31	27	-13%	24	-23%
	Vitamin B6	330	27	-92%	18	-95%
Strawberries	Calcium	21	18	-14%	12	-43%
	Vitamin C	60	13	-78%	8	-87%

Table 2: Nutritional value of fruits and vegetables in 1985-1996-2002 - Geigy.

Today, there is a scientific concordance in favor of the taking of food supplements, even in the context of a quality diet. Finally, there are the epidemiological studies, all of which lead to a deficiency of at least 4 nutrients in the majority of populations in industrialized countries: vitamin D, magnesium, zinc and omega 3 fatty acids.

The case of vitamin D is particularly shocking: one estimates that thousands of deaths would be avoided with a simple vitamin D supplement. However, despite all the research and studies, the daily recommendation guideline in the US and Europe remains ridiculously low (on average 400-800 IU or 10-20 micrograms per day).

"Bioidentical hormone treatments are complete nonsense."

Another grievance that is frequently heard with that of premature aging. Again, this statement is not scientific.

Naysayers of anti-aging medicine would be better off minding their own business rather than criticizing. After all, people who live in glass houses shouldn't throw stones. To take the example of a well-known chemical molecule sildenafil (Viagra®), only a double-blind study was carried out before it was marketed by Pfizer. For statins, it's not much better, their designer Rory Collins from the University of Oxford, has even recently admitted to having deliberately neglected examining the side effects, so convinced that there were benefits of these molecules among patients with high cholesterol levels (27).

In reality, anti-aging medicine is an "evidence-based medicine", supported by thousands of studies done on the effects of the same bio-hormone for decades. We will see below with the "creatine business" how bad beliefs can lead to misinformation at the highest level of the state.

"THE CREATINE BUSINESS" EXAMPLE: HOW FRANCE BECAME A WORLD -WIDE LAUGHING STOCK

In Polynesia, where I have lived for around thirty years, the regulations in force concerning dietary supplements are often modeled on French regulations.

This is not always a good idea, as we will see with the creatine example. The complete history of its ban can be found in the book by Thierry Souccar: *Santé, Mensonges et Propagande* but I will try to summarize here as the book is written in French and it is a peculiar case.

Creatine is a natural substance present in meat and used by a number of athletes to enhance their performance. It was sold freely in a number of countries until, 23rd January 2001, the international press released a statement from the AFFSA (French Food Safety Agency) decreeing the carcinogenicity of creatine. Indeed, although not on the list of doping products, the French government circles decided to counter the opinion of the International Olympic Committee and pronounce its ban. This was not easy because at that point, creatine was circulating freely in Europe, and a member country cannot ban it unless it proves the product is dangerous.

This opinion by the AFFSA has stunned many experts including Professor Jacques Poortmans from the University of Brussels, who has published many studies on creatine, without ever mentioning a carcinogenic risk. He claims to be "blown away" by the statements of AFFSA, relayed by the US agency Reuters.

In reality, the "evidence" of AFFSA lies in a misinterpretation of an article by Dr. Markus Wyss (Basel, Switzerland) entitled "Creatine and creatinine metabolism". Wyss says he is "enormously astonished" by the conclusions of the experts from the AFFSA and adds that they did not read his text correctly. Indeed, the production of AHA (Aromatic Heterocyclic Anions) can be formed during the cooking of meat containing creatine, but the formation of AHA in the body from the direct ingestion of creatine has never been demonstrated. On the contrary, creatine is, according to Markus Wyss, a "potential anticancer agent".

In fact, to meet their goal, the AFFSA "experts" have selected an isolated study showing the in-vitro formation of AHA at 37°C, and neglected the mass studies that prove otherwise.

Coincidentally, this opinion of the AFFSA fell at the moment when companies marketing creatine, like RCS, are sued before the Court of Appeal of Anger (victorious in the First Instance) and where the company INKO lodges an appeal against France before the European Court of Justice. The same company lodged a complaint against the then Minister of Health, Marie George Buffet, who accused INKO of "incitement to doping".

Nowadays, creatine is sold in all pharmacies and drugstores and the case may make you smile, if it had not had to reproduce with other supplements like taurine.

Indeed, taurine has been banned in Polynesia for a few years, by bureaucrats from the Health Directorate, probably influenced by its presence in certain energy drinks whose safety has been controversial. However, this antioxidant amino acid produced by the liver in the human body has demonstrated numerous positive effects on health, particularly of the nervous and muscular system. It can be taken at a dosage of up to 3 grams per day without any harmful effects.

We now know that taurine helps magnesium to enter into the cell (with vitamin B6), and the best magnesium supplements on the market contain it.

We will see later that I also use it as an anti-DHT agent - dihydrotestosterone - (with another amino acid, lysine) as part of the androgenic alopecia control protocol.

WHICH SUPPLEMENTS AND WHERE TO FIND THEM?

You have two options: go into your local pharmacy or order them on the internet. The majority of healthcare professional will formally advise against the second option, alleging that products sold on the internet are not controlled.

So what is the best option?

To find out, the nutritionists from the site www.lanutrition.fr have written numerous fact sheets on the benefits of vitamins and multivitamins.

On the podium are brands sold exclusively on the internet, such as Supersmart, Nutriting, Cellinov. Products sold in pharmacies generally suffer from poor formulation, with pro oxidants such as copper or iron, synthetic vitamin E lacking all tocopherol isomers, not to mention sweeteners or preservatives.

My experience:

There is not one brand that is the best for all vitamins and minerals. Always look at the composition, knowing that european products are generally under dosed with vitamin D for legislative reasons. For omega 3, always look at the EPA/DHA fatty acid content, as it should be at least 1g per day, and make sure they are checked for their heavy metal content by IFOS. Personally, I often buy from a US pharmaceutical grade brand such as Jarrow.

For hormones such as DHEA or pregnenolone, the laboratory dosages that I have been able to carry out always show a good content of product in the capsules, including premium brands like Vitacost. The important thing for a good follow-up, is to stay with the same brands over a few months, and always carry out these analyses in the same laboratory.

Here are the essentials, i.e. those which most of us are deficient in:

OMEGA 3 FATTY ACIDS (fish oil).

The ratio of omega 3/ omega 6 is very unfavorable in our current diet, due to meat and fish farms fed on cereal, and industrial food. This results in a state of chronic inflammation. Unless you eat 3 boxes of sardines a week, this dietary supplement is an essential part of an anti-aging program. Know that there is an inverse relationship between fish consumption and the risk of breast cancer. The risk reduction is around 30% for women who consume the most fish.

MAGNESIUM

A common deficiency. 25% of women and 20% of men suffer from magnesium deficiency (less than 2/3 of recommended nutritional intake). Like zinc, this element is needed for several hundred enzymatic reactions (at least 600 according to researchers). It is sold in many forms, and not all are equal. Along with those with the highest bioavailability are the citrate, bisglycinate and aspartate forms. The chloride form, one of the least expensive sold in pharmacies, although of high bioavailability is to be discouraged. Indeed, the chloride ions make it acidifying for the organism, and we will see further the importance of preserving a neutral or slightly alkaline medium. It is also probably the acidifying property of magnesium chloride that makes it effective to fight against certain bacterial or even viral infections. But a long-term acidic organism makes a breeding ground for cancer, as shown by Nobel Prize winner Dr Otto Warburg in the 1930s. We will see how to handle all of the this with the PRAL index of foods.

In addition, magnesium chloride is a laxative!

The best forms are in citrate or chelated glycinate form, combined with vitamin B6 and taurine for easy absorption at cell level.

It is the anti-stress element par excellence, it has a soothing and muscle-relaxing effect that makes it interesting to take in the afternoon or evening. In addition, it limits the rise of cortisol. Please note however, that some authors say that it can interfere with the absorption of thyroid hormones: it is an additional reason to take it at the end of the day.

ZINC

It is a catalyst of many biological reactions and its rate can drop when over-exerted. There is also a frequency deficiency with age too. One can measure out this element in the laboratory. The prostate contains a large quantity, and this element is essential for its health. Zinc boosts immunity, and is good for skin and hair. It plays a fundamental role in combination with melatonin and selenium during sleep in order to maintain good immune health (13). The famous researcher Walter Pierpaoli, one of my teachers, has developed a melatonin associated with zinc and selenium, and excipients allowing its release around 3am, when the catch takes place between 22h and 23h.

Please note, an excess of zinc can cause copper deficiency. It should not exceed 50mg per day in supplementation.

"Rubozinc", a commonly prescribed form available in pharmacies, contains gluten and lactose.

VITAMIN D3 (cholecalciferol): for whom? why? what can we expect?

Vitamin D is not a vitamin

In reality, vitamin D is a steroid hormone, such as pregnenolone, DHEA, estrogen, progesterone, cortisol or testosterone. This means that vitamin D and cholesterol are linked. Cholesterol levels that are too low will have an impact on the synthesis of vitamin D like other steroid hormones.

Vitamin D is not only responsible for fighting against rickets, as many doctors still believe. It is the essential cofactor of numerous reactions within the body. Without Vitamin D, thyroid hormones cannot enter the cell and immunity deteriorates leaving you at a higher risk of diseases like cancer. Vitamin D-deficient adolescents have less methylated DNA than others, and this translates into an increased risk of cancer, atherosclerosis, or autoimmune disease.

What are the recommendations?

We are on the brink of a sanitary scandal. The vast majority of France's population are deficient and official recommended intake - which varies depending on the country - was ridiculously low in France (400 IU: this dosage does not optimize the level of vitamin D3 in the blood). In 2016, the European agency revised the dosage and increased it up to 600 IU. Two years later, France finally aligned with these recommendations. According to the health monitoring institute, 80% of French people suffer from a vitamin D deficiency. Indeed, the latitude of

our country does not allow a sufficient amount of exposure to the sun all year round. This deficiency is a problem for laboratory standards, which are statistical standards, as we will see later. Today, vitamin D is the most studied supplement in the scientific community, and for good reason. Its role has such an impact on immunity that it is estimated that thousands of lives could be spared by a slight adjustment of vitamin D. More than just a vitamin, it is a pro-hormone that has shown its protective role against cancer from 50 ng/ml, and an important role against osteoporosis (14). It also has an effect on autoimmune diseases and is able to regulate intestinal permeability. It was the Garland brothers who made it famous, demonstrating that melanoma is not directly linked to sun exposure, contrary to popular belief. Their study of cancer in the US army showed that against all odds, sailors were surprisingly not the most affected by melanoma despite their frequent exposure to the sun. The most affected were in fact submariners who do not see natural light for weeks, sometimes months.
Their study demonstrated the importance of regular sun exposure, adapted to the skin's phenotype, in order to maintain a good level of vitamin D.

According to a large analysis (Garland 2007, 2 studies with 1760 patients) the diminution of the risk of cancer is 50% from 52 ng/ml, which corresponds to a dosage of less than 4000 UI per day, largely superior to the recommendations from the National Academy of Sciences (2000 UI). Garland (2009) suggests that 60,000 new cases of cancer could be prevented if the dosage of vitamin D was adjusted between 40 and 50 ng/ml which is around 2000 UI per day. I recommend to carry out a laboratory test, and to supplement at a dosage of between 60 and 80 ng/ml of blood.

Whether you are a pro-swimmer or a professional surfer, supplements concern everybody.

What advantages do supplements bring?

They adjust the level of Vitamin D in your blood between 60 and 80ng/ml allowing you to decrease your risk of:

- ✓ 50% of heart attacks
- ✓ 80% of multiple sclerosis
- ✓ 83% of flu
- ✓ 50% osteoporosis fractures
- ✓ 71% type 1 diabetes
- ✓ 83% prostate cancer
- ✓ 80% colon cancer
- ✓ 50% leukemia
- ✓ 65 to 75% of pancreatic, bladder and kidney cancer
- ✓ 63% of asthma

In order to start the supplementation, begin with a dosage of 75 UI/kg of weight and adjust according to the laboratory result. Personally, although I live in a tropical country (I expose myself to little sun), I take around 6000 UI per day. There is no toxicity below 10,000 UI per day. Plus, there is a regulating mechanism at skin level depending on sun exposure, so no need to worry! The strong doses that doctors often prescribe, valid for several weeks in the form of vials, are not recommended. It is better to take it daily so it is more consistent with the natural synthesis of vitamin D that our skin receives from sun exposure. Zyma D is inexpensive in pharmacies, and its formulation in the form of drops allows an exact adjustment of the dosage (1 drop = 300 IU). To prevent osteoporosis, it is advisable to couple it with vitamin K2 MK7. Please note: people who are undergoing anti-coagulant treatment (AVK) can not take vitamin K.

MARK SISSON'S PALEOLITHIC MODEL.

In the 1980s, the athlete Mark Sisson popularized what he calls the Paleolithic model and published an eponymous bestseller in his French translation.

More than a diet, this model is a way of life, based on unprocessed, low carbohydrate diets, and how to be more active.

Scientifically recognized today, this way of life seems the most effective way to preserve our endocrine glands and sustain a normal weight. Part of the reason for its success is that it involves no calorie counting - you can still eat well!

The Paleolithic diet is based on the fact that the human genome has hardly evolved between the Paleolithic era and today. On the other hand, the diet changed considerably after the industrial and agricultural revolution, but not over a long enough period for our genes to adapt. This diet is quite similar to Dr. Seignalet, who first highlighted the link between intestinal permeability and autoimmune diseases.

Here are the 12 basic rules:

1. **Eliminate products rich in carbohydrates:**

For your health and also your children's, breakfast cereals should only be found in one place: the bin! These are ultra-processed products, extruded, blown up, heated at high temperatures, stratospheric glycemic index and all the claims on the package are ridiculous. You will notice that there are many of these types of product in the supermarket. It is because the sales margins are enormous and cost little to manufacture.

Sodas, pastries, ice creams, sausages, bread are all processed products that should be eliminated or strongly limited.

To rid your body of sweet products, it takes at least 3 difficult weeks; but it's worth the effort. The daily consumption of sugar results in a decrease in sensitivity of insulin receptors by secretion of this hormone from the pancreas, otherwise known as … diabetes! (Type 2) Plus, the pathologies that come with diabetes lead to premature aging.

Remember that allopathic medicine can not cure diabetes!

Beware of the multitude of hidden sugars that are in modern diets. It is easy to find them by consulting the table of glycemic indexes. Indeed, the idea of "fast release" and "slow release" sugars has been outdated for a long time, even if we still hear about it!

All foods are classified according to an index of 100 which is based on elevated glucose levels after glucose intake. The higher the index, the more you have to limit your food. A high index is more than 70 whereas a low index is less than 55 which is more favorable.

Beer, white bread, low quality white rice all have a high index even though they do not have a sweet taste. White bread has a higher index than that of sucrose (white sugar)!

2. Eat the right fats.

Today we are witnessing the return of fat that has long been demonized by the sugar industry and its lobbies. Following the false recommendations from the

PNNS (National Nutrition and Health Program), there has been a veritable epidemic of obesity in recent decades.

Fortunately, we have now rediscovered the benefits of fat in a ketogenic diet to fight against cancer. We also saw the return to grace of coconut oil, interesting for its lauric acid content and medium-chain triglycerides.

By contrast, there is now a decrease in the amount of omega 3 we can access. Present in wild meat and fish, nowadays we almost find more in livestock products that we consume every day. I recommend, if you have the opportunity, to consume hen eggs raised with linseed, rich in omega 3. Also consume rapeseed oil and small fatty fish like sardines for their low levels of heavy metal contaminants.

Omega 3 has such a long list of benefits that you would think it's a miracle food. It is one of the cornerstones of a Mediterranean diet. By improving the communication between the cells and their walls, it facilitates learning. Deficiencies cause attention disorders in children.

They reduce inflammation by playing on cytokines and TNF alpha and compete with omega 6 pro-inflammatory drugs. They facilitate recovery, reduce muscle soreness after exercise, joint pain and promote muscle growth. No doubt the Greek god Poseidon consumed a lot of it!

They lower the level of triglycerides and help normalize the lipid balance. The researcher Michel de Lorgeril has studied their effects as a replacement for statins, an expensive and controversial treatment because of its side effects and risk/benefit ratio is doubtful.

They could help prevent cancer, including breast, colon and prostate.

They would also be effective in rheumatoid arthritis and ankylosing spondylitis.

3. Eat enough protein!

With age, the body loses muscle mass every year. This is called sarcopenia and starts at the age of 30 at 3-8% per year. The process accelerates at 50 years old and leads, when severe, to an increase in morbidity and mortality (11).

It is one of the reasons that it is important to eat enough good-quality protein, taking the majority of your intake at the start of the day. Why reduce the intake of protein in the evening? Because they slow down the functioning of the thyroid gland during the night and the transformation of the hormone T4 into T3 (the active form). Not ideal to keep your figure in check.

Macronutrient essential, the recommended intake does not exceed 1g per kg of weight per day in adulthood but I think it should be increased if you do more sport.

Be careful however, proteins are acidifying for the body, their PRAL index is unfavorable. To alkalize the body, it is necessary to compensate with a good amount of fruit and vegetables or even consider a potassium supplement. It is indeed the intake of potassium contained in fruits and vegetables that maintains an alkaline environment. See the PRAL table of foods.

Animal protein or vegetables?
Both sources are good. When it comes to protein powder, for eager athletes, one finds that next to the traditional whey protein or the whey isolate (lactose-free whey protein), a whole range of vegetable proteins. Alas, they do not all have an amino-gram as interesting as whey

protein. It seems that the best among the plant forms is hemp protein … if you can swallow it!

4. Cook food at a low temperature.

Although the raw diet has its followers, some authors think that the evolution of man is due to the cooking of food, making its nutrients more assimilable for our bodies.

However, cooking at high temperatures causes the Maillard reaction, as I said above. This glycation of proteins releases toxic substances. That's why barbecuing food is not recommended, it is better to slow cook or steam.

Personally, I cook my breakfast eggs on the cooker at a minimum temperature, with olive or coconut oil.

5. Fruits and vegetables in every meal!

Anything that can't be found in nature is not paleo. So throw out your dauphinois potatoes and rediscover the flavor of vegetables cooked in water with olive oil… and all the spices you want. For fruits, the less-sweet ones are better, such as berries, pears and dried fruits which we tend to leave out of our meals.

6. Lift weights, sprint from time to time, walk barefoot.

Yes, movement is life. Contrary to popular belief, osteoarthritis is not a wearing of the joints and becomes worse the less you move.

The benefits of bodybuilding in anti-aging medicine are well established: it effectively combats sarcopenia, the metabolic syndrome. By its very nature (not successively and for a limited time), it is one sporting activity that boosts the growth hormone the most, which is crucial as one ages.

The ideal session should not exceed one hour, beyond which other, less desirable, catabolic hormones will take over such as cortisol and catecholamines.

Walking barefoot helps the body maintain balance. The total proprioception of the foot is ideal as well as shock absorption without the use of shoes as they encourage us to walk on our heels.

7. Earn your carbs.

Indeed, the amount of carbohydrates you consume must be in proportion to your physical activity. Periods without physical activity do not require a significant carbohydrate intake; otherwise fat intake is guaranteed! Remember it's the carbohydrates that make you fat not the fat as information campaigns have been "teaching" us for the past 40 years. Of course, when it comes to carbohydrates, it will always be those of fruits and starchy foods. In my country, sweet potato and taro are an ideal source as they are rich in nutrients. In any case, if you have doubts, consult the glycemic index tables, remembering that taste is not a good indicator in this area. Indeed, who would have thought that puffed rice cakes which are abundant in the organic aisles, have a stratospheric glycemic index and are capable of ruining your diet?

8. Make small meals every 3 hours... or not!

In addition to the three main meals, you can have a snack mid-morning, mid-afternoon and after sport. By snack, I do not mean a cereal bar packed with sugar and no nutritional value. Instead, opt for a protein snack, almonds, organic fruit that is slightly sweet. By continuing with this habit, your stomach will not get bigger and you will control your insulin secretion better. Remember that any peak in insulin causes a hypoglycaemic reaction in the following hours. This explains the well-known "slump" after eating a heavy meal. Moreover, by eating little and often, you are constantly supplying your body with nutrients. However, if you're not hungry, don't only eat because it's a time of day that you usually associate with eating. We all descend from hunter gatherers who did not eat three times a day at specific times! Our bodies are not made for that, unless we want to be permanently bloated.

9. Eat from a small plate.

This recommendation may seem far-fetched but studies have shown that over the years the size of our plates have increased and so have our portions. It has been shown that by using a small plate, we are inclined to eat less.

10. Examine everything you eat and ask yourself the big question.

What is this question you ask? It is: What will this food bring me?

I mean, what is its nutritional value? Does it still contain vitamins, minerals, proteins, fibre and good fats?

You will quickly start to realize that white rice does not bring much value compared to quinoa or sweet potato. You will also get a better understanding of why processed products are not good for the body.

By focusing on foods with high nutritional value, you have the secret to achieve and maintain a slim and toned body whatever your age.

11. Take probiotics.

Yes, the latest studies all show that the intestinal flora of people suffering from obesity is different from that of slim and athletic athletes. You can change this flora according to your diet. As such, I recommend brewer's years and sauerkraut for their high content of microorganisms.

12. Chew more!

Eating soft foods makes you fat, and the modern diet requires less and less chewing. Mashed potatoes, fruit juices, minced meats. Mastication allows the production of saliva, whose alkalizing and protective role in the oesophagus avoids gastroesophageal reflux. In addition, this essential mastication step allows better management of appetite and satiety - two physiological states controlled by two hormones, ghrelin and leptin. One more reason to eat paleo, the least modified possible.

TABLE OF GLYCEMIC INDEX:

Heightened GI (>70)	Moderate GI (between 56 and 69)	Low GI (<55)
Fruits		
Dates: 103	Fresh apricots: 57 Melon: 67 Cherries: 63 Papaya: 56 Ripe banana: 65 Dried figs: 61 Dried raisins: 64 Pineapple: 59 Apricots in syrup: 64 Peaches in syrup: 58	Fresh apple: 38 Dried apricots: 30 Grapefruit: 25 Grapes: 53 Unripe banana: 52 Kiwi: 53 Pear: 38 Orange: 42 Apple juice with no added sugar: 44 Grapefruit juice with no sugar added: 50 Tomato juice: 38
Oleaginous Fruits		
		Pecan nuts: 10 Salted cashew nuts: 22 Salted, toasted peanuts: 14
Vegetables		
		All vegetables have a low GI often very low (<15)

		Raw carrots: 16 Cooked carrots: 47
Legumes		
		Dried green lentils cooked in water: 48 Red lentils: 26 Tinned lentils: 48 Dried chick peas cooked in water: 28 Peas: 41
Soya and derived products		
		Soya milk enriched in calcium: 36 Soya yoghurt with fruits: 50 Tofu: Contains no carbohydrates.
Potatoes		
Roast potatoes: 95 Instant mashed potato: 83 Peeled, boiled potatoes: 78 New potatoes with skin, boiled: 78 Fries: 82	Steamed potatoes with skin: 65	Baked potato: 46 Crisps (chips US): 54

Cereals and derived products		
White baguette: 95 White baguette (60g) with chocolate spread (20g): 72 White sandwich bread: 70 Whole wheat bread: 71 White toast: 68 Waffles: 76 Apricot tartlet: 71 Kellogg's Cornflakes: 77 Kellogg's Corn Pops: 80 Kellogg's Rice Krispies: 82 Kelloggs's Smacks: 71 Instant oats: 82 Rice cakes: 85 Quick-cooking rice: 87	Wholemeal loaf: 65 White baguette (60g) with butter (10g) and raspberry jam (20g): 62 Croissant: 67 Chocolate digestive: 56 Traditional rolled outs: 59 Kellogg's Special K: 56 White rice cooked in water: 64 Basmati rice: 58 Gnocchi: 68 Polenta: 68	Wholewheat bread: 49 Pumpernickel (German black bread): 50 Dry butter biscuit: 50 Belvita chocolate breakfast biscuits: 42 Kellogg's All Bran: 34 Natural Muesli: 49 Macaroni: 47 Vermicelli: 35 Cooked spaghetti 10-15min: 44 Mixed grains cooked for 10min: 50 Brown rice: 50 Pizza Hut: 36
Sodas, drinks		
	Coca-cola: 63 Fanta orange: 68 Bière: 66	
Sugar, sweets, snacks		

Glucose: 100 Sweets: 78	White sugar (table sugar): 68 Chocolate bar Mars: 68 Milk chocolate: 64 Mixed commercial honey: 62 Jams: 66	Fructose: 10 Snickers: 41 Twix: 44 M&M's: 33 Maple syrup: 54 Reduced- sugar Apricot jam: 55 Nutella:33
Milk Products		
	Sweetened condensed milk: 61	Low-fat fruit yoghurts: 26 Full-fat milk: 27 Semi-skimmed milk: 30 Ice cream: 47
Meat, eggs, seafood		
These foods have a low glycemic index because they contain little or no carbohydrates.		

THE PRAL INDEX OF 80 FOODS:

It is quite simple to read: any food above 0 is acidifying. This is the case with protein, dairy products and cereals in general. Anything below 0 is alkaline.

Food	PRAL (mEq/100g)
Fish	
Cod	9.9
Haddock	10.6
Smoked herring	12.4
Trout	13.5
Meat	
Beef	11.3
Roast chicken with skin.	14.6
Frankfurt sausage	9.8
Cooked pork	13.3
Salami	7.7
Roast turkey with skin	15.6
Veal escalope	18.7
Cereal products	
Wholewheat bread	6.1

White bread	4.2
Corn flakes	2.8
Egg noodles	6.4
Oats cooked in water	1.7
Wholegrain rice	2.2
White rice	1.6
White flour	9.1
Wholewheat flour	10.2
Milk products	
Camembert	13
Cheddar	26.4
Gouda	20
Vanilla ice cream	0.5
Whole milk	0.1
Parmesan	27.8
Fruit yoghurt	-0.4
Eggs	
Chicken's eggs	7.2
Fruits	
Apple with skin	-1.9
Apricot	-4.3

Banana	-6.9
Blackcurrant	-5.2
Cherry	-3
Kiwi	-5.6
Orange	-3
Peach	-3.1
Pear	-2.1
Pineapple	-2.3
Grape	-6.1
Strawberry	-2.5
Watermelon	-2
Unbleached nuts	-2.4
Nuts	5.6
Vegetables	
Asparagus	-0.4
Broccoli	-3.6
Raw carrot	-5.7
Raw cauliflower	-4.4
Cooked celery	-5.5
Cucumber	-2.4
Aubergine	-2

Cooked pepper	-1.6
Lettuce	-2.2
Mushrooms	-3.6
Raw onion	-2
Potato	-5.2
Radish	-4.4
Spinach	-10.3
Tomato	-5.3
Courgette	-4.3
Legumes	
Green beans	-2.8
Lentils	2.1
Tinned peas	1.4
Drinks	
Blonde beer	-0.1
Coca-cola	0.3
Hot chocolate	-0.4
Espresso coffee	-4.2
Red wine	-2.2
Tea	-0.8
Dry white wine	-1.2

Lemon juice	-2.4
Apple juice	-2
Orange juice	-2.9
Grape juice	-1.9
Tomato juice	-4.1
Sweet products	
Chocolate milk	0.7
Honey	-0.9
Fruitcake	1.2
Apricot jam	-1.5
White sugar	0

Source: lanutrition.fr (translated into English)

METABOLIC SYNDROME OR « SYNDROME X »

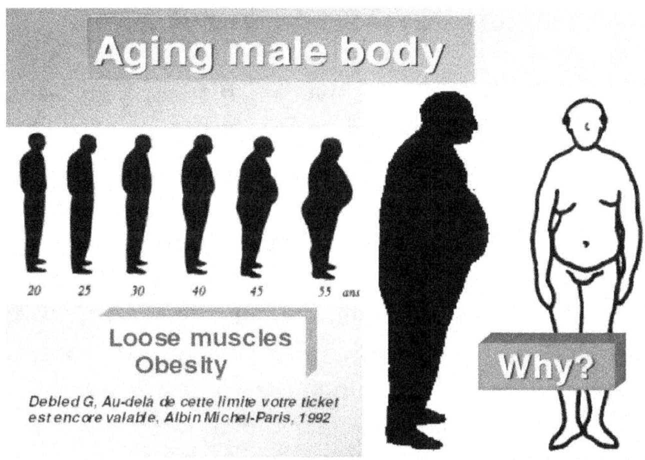

The metabolic syndrome or syndrome X is defined by a progressive decrease in insulin sensitivity, an increase in the ratio of hip circumference/chest circumference, a deterioration of lipid parameters, sometimes accompanied by hypertension. These signs, which one could associate with a jovial character and a comfortable lifestyle in the person who is affected, hide a much darker reality. In fact, the risk of stroke and cardiovascular disease are greatly increased. More precisely, the cardiovascular risk is multiplied by three.

In men, it is the belly that gets bigger, favored by a slow and inexorable drop in sex hormone levels. In addition to adipose tissue that is linked to increased estrogen levels, it is not uncommon to see gynecomastia (swelling of the breast tissue).

Basically, this is what I call the heron syndrome, because it is often accompanied by a visible muscular loss in thighs.

In menopausal women, cardiovascular disease is similar to men's risk because of the drop in estrogen.

Moreover, it is not uncommon to see higher estrogen in overweight men over 45 than in menopausal women. We will see later that estrogen in men is becoming more and more suspected as a cause of benign prostatic hyperplasia.

From the front, the body seems to resemble a pear shape, and many physical signs of aging begin to appear: fatigue with little activity, thinking becomes less clear, the face is paler, hair loses volume or starts to fall out by accelerating the degradation of testosterone to dihydrotestosterone (DHT) under the action of enzyme 5 alpha reductase. Size also decreases due to bone decalcification and growth hormone deficiency combined with lower testosterone. If nothing is done at the dietary and/or hormonal level, osteoporosis sets in, the lipid balance continues to deteriorate, and aging accelerates.

DO YOUR OWN SHOPPING!

It's time to change the contents of your pantry!

It goes without saying that you cannot change your diet overnight but instead use the Japanese method of "small steps".

For my part, I only changed my breakfast in the first few months and that was a big step!

I used to eat sugary cereals with no milk, no fruit, sometimes coffee and toast with jam and juice. This type of breakfast that is commonly known as "continental" in hotels, is not the way to go. It lacks a variation of nutrients, antioxidants and is full of sugar. At the age of 45, it caused the start of metabolic syndrome with a slight increase in triglycerides. Yet, I still thought I was safe from any lipid balance degradation with my rates already being quite low in adolescence. My doctor had told me that high triglycerides = sugar but I had not yet figured out how to find the hidden sugars and I did not know about the concept of glycemic index.

Anyway, with my health deteriorating (joint pain in particular), I decided to change my breakfast and it has hardly changed since. Here it is:

- 2 to 3 fried eggs (organic if possible) or an omelette cooked slowly with coconut or olive oil, lots of turmeric and pepper.

- Buckwheat flakes softened with with boiling water and then accompanied with almond milk and often, a teaspoon of locally-sourced honey.

- Green tea

- Some fruit containing little sugar (not banana)

- Vitamin supplements, fatty acids, bioidentical hormones (see further on)

As you can see, bread and cows milk don't feature in this recipe. There is no longer any fruit juice but a large glass of water to swallow the supplements.

The problem with milk:
- **Lactose in milk has never been well digested by the body as well as its protein, caseine.**
- **It is an acidifying food, meaning that it has a detrimental effect on calcium absorption.**
- **Milk increases the intestinal permeability (such as gluten and potatoes..) which over a period of time can cause auto immune diseases.**
- **Milk contains hormones and growth factors which are used to make the cows bigger. In men, it seems to enlarge the prostate, as professor Joyeux humorously stated.**
- **In Chinese medicine, milk is classified as "humidifying" and it does not recommend it as a good source of calcium.**
- **Scandinavians, who consume a lot of milk, suffer from more fractures compared to Asians, who do not consume as much (12).**

Bread is a processed product that has no place in a paleo diet. Worse, bread or white bread are insulin bombs that can ruin your efforts to lose weight in a short period of time. Finally, modern wheat is an O.G.M toxin that has doubled the number of chromosomes (compared to ancestral wheat) to make it produce the maximum amount of gluten. This protein with little nutritional value increases the problem of intestinal permeability and turns your digestive tract into a colander. In doing so, the gut passes molecules that it should usually block. This produces antibodies in the blood, which can attach to some of your organs and destroy them little by little (14).

I've always been a big pasta and bread eater until I was 45 years old until I learnt about the probable origin of my Hashimoto's thyroiditis, an autoimmune disease, discovered at 32 years old - the same time as my two melanomas. We will see later on that there is a link between these two pathologies.

Here is a typical list that can be adapted according to where you live. We must always focus on short circuits: avoid food from distant sources, whose carbon footprint is often catastrophic and vitamin intake often low due to transport.

Proteins:
- Rump steak or tenderloin beef
- Chicken breast
- Salmon steak
- Organic eggs if possible, from hens fed on flax seeds
- Small fish (sardine, mackerel)
- For people who live in tropical countries: lagoon fish (without ciguatera)
- Limit pelagic fish intake due to accumulation of heavy metals

Carbohydrates:
- Basmati rice (moderate glycemic index)
- Mashed potato
- Quinoa

- Lentils
- Saracen flour, from coconuts
- Oats and Saracen

Fats:

- All dried fruits: almonds, hazelnuts, walnuts… the brazil nut is equally interesting for it selenium content
- coconut oil, coconut milk
- avocado
- Cold-pressed virgin olive oil. Avoid sources such as "European union oil blend"

Fruits and vegetables:

There is so much choice: carrots, courgettes, aubergines, broccoli, spinach, white onions, garlic, bananas (not overripe), frozen red fruits or fresh, lemons, kiwi, pear, papaya, mango… choose fruit that is in season in your region. Apples are usually the most treated with pesticides (about fifteen treatments for this fruit!) and grapes.

Various and spices:
Organic green tea is rich in epigallocatechins (antioxidant) in its leaves, bags, Macha powder or Sencha for amateurs.
Spices are alkalizing, anti inflammatory (turmeric, ginger, clove), hypoglycemic (Sri Lankan cinnamon), get involved!

THE HORMONE DIET

Food influences the endocrine gland much more than is believed. Insulin has long been accepted as a fact as well as other hormones.

Yet, we will see some simple rules that can be applied to stay slim. Dr Thierry Hertoghe, a world specialist in anti-aging medicine, has written a book "The Hormone Diet".

In short, know that the hunter-gatherer diet, or Paleolithic, is the one that keeps your endocrine glands in check the best.

Conversely, hormonal deficiencies can be revealed by examining how the patient is eating. For example, a person with hypothyroidism will be tired when they wake up in the morning and drink coffee in order to wake them up. In turn, coffee stimulates the adrenal glands, which will eventually run out in the long run. Thus, cortisol and DHEA deficiency are not uncommon in poorly-treated hypothyroid patients.

What to eat to stimulate your thyroid?

Fruits and more fruits!

A few years ago, I was eating so much fruit (mostly mangoes), that I had hyperthyroidism and had to lower my thyroxin intake. Obviously, this level of consumption is not advised long term but its good to know you can wake up a lazy thyroid with a proper diet.

And for growth hormones?

Stop all sugar intake after 5pm.

Take 2 grams of glutamine at bedtime or a MK677 secretagogue (adults only).

Indeed, there is an antinomic relationship between insulin and the growth hormone (HGH), and any late consumption of sugar slows its secretion.

Also, avoid caffeine and increase your protein intake during the day.

How can elderly men limit their estrogen?

Estrogen, known as a "female" sex hormone, contains three hormones (estrone (E1), estradiol (E2) and estriol(E3)) that play a vital role in both women and men at cardiovascular level and bone level. During menopause, the risk of stroke in women is similar to that of men, due to the decline in estrogen. It is not uncommon for overweight men to have higher levels of estrogen than menopausal women of the same age. In addition to the problem of gynecomastia, excess estrogen in humans are increasingly suspected as the cause of prostate cancer, which then grows under the influence of dihydrotestosterone (DHT).

Avoid alcohol, sugar, coffee and sausages that activate aromatase, the enzyme that breaks down testosterone into estrogen. We will also see that this conversion takes place in the adipose tissue, and that limiting weight makes it easier to control the level of estrogen. Soybeans, whose isoflavones are phytoestrogens, should also be avoided. However, these may be of interest to menopausal women who are not taking hormone therapy as they limit the unpleasant symptoms of menopause.

What to eat in the evening to stay slim?

You should limit the amount of proteins in your evening meal, because these slow down the conversion of thyroid hormone T4 into T3 (the active form). On the other hand, we will see later that melatonin taken before bedtime aids this conversion, as well as the secretion of all hormones except cortisol, which decreases.

CALORIE RESTRICTION AND LONGEVITY

All studies in animals have shown the effect of caloric restriction on longevity. On the Mediline portal, there are nearly 3000 studies on this subject.

Intermittent fasting produces similar effects and is also being used more and more by athletes.

All of these techniques should only be done under medical supervision.

The Paleolithic model also allows fasting, as observed sometimes in the tribes of hunter-gatherers.

Certain supplements including **resveratrol**, a polyphenol from the family of stilbenes, synthesized by plants is able to mimic the caloric restriction on a biological level. It particularly protects against the decrease of the number hepatic mitochondria induced by a high calorie diet.

Metformin, well known for the treatment of diabetes, induces a marked increase in the longevity of animals (15). Its "off-label" use for anti-aging purposes requires further study.

There is a natural substance, **berberine**, whose hypoglycemic properties are at least equal or superior to those of metformin. Alas, I do not know any studies about berberine and longevity. It is a shame that berberine is not regularly recommended endocrinologists. However, qualified doctors in functional and nutritional medicine, who are becoming more numerous in France, advise this supplement.

THE SECRET OF THE MITOCHONDRIA?

More and more researchers believe that the key to longevity lies in the mitochondria, "the power station" of the cell. In fact, the latest studies have caused a buzz in the scientific community, including those on **NAD+**. **Nicotinamide Adenine Dinucleotide (or NAD)** is a valuable cofactor in all of the body's cells. This natural product, and therefore unpatentable, is a derivative of vitamin B3, or niacin. Aging is accompanied by a decline in NAD, hence the idea from researchers to test its supplementation in animals. The results, while very encouraging, can not be extrapolated to humans and require further study. Unfortunately, NAD is produced and manufactured by the company NIAGEN, which has succeeded in patenting this molecule, yet natural, and sells it for a high price. A good alternative at a modest price is **niacinamide** and several studies have shown its beneficial effects on the skin, including a reduction of about 30% in the risk of basal cell carcinoma, the most common skin cancer in elderly people (16). The dose used for this purpose is 1g per day. In my experience niacinamide, has allowed me to reduce and even virtually stop new onsets of basal cell carcinoma, at a time of my life when the condition of my skin was starting to become very worrisome. As we will see later, hormones are also beneficial for the cutaneous tissue, including thyroid hormones, whose optimization of my treatment (an addition of T3 to the already prescribed T4) has undoubtably positively influenced the resolution of my skin problems. To be clear, I stopped niacinamide supplementation for two months, and I unfortunately saw the resurgence of a "baso" on my forehead. So I took niacinamide at a dose of 500g morning and evening. In some people, niacinamide can cause a hot flush which may be uncomfortable, but there are also "flush free" forms available.

Coenzyme Q10 also plays a key role in the mitochondria, the body synthesizes less with age, and supplementation has shown a protective effect in cardiovascular disease. **It should be taken systematically by all those who are on statins,** these very controversial anti-cholesterol molecules which also lower the rate of coenzyme Q10. All anti-aging doctors take it! (see further anti-aging doctor programs).

PART 3

HORMONES: A SYMPHONIC ORCHESTRA

Italian researcher Walter Pierpaoli, an expert of the pineal gland and melatonin, wrote that hormones act like a symphonic orchestra in our bodies. It's a beautiful image and illustrates the interactions that occur between hormones. Often, treatment with a single hormone will give disappointing results, or even show side effects, as is often the case when we take cortisol, for example. Even worse, synthetic cortisone, without adding DHEA compensates for the catabolic effects of cortisol. Similarly, anti-aging physicians rarely prescribe DHEA on its own in women, without taking care to add female sex hormones, to limit the the potentially virilizing effect of DHEA. It is important to know all these interactions. Even melatonin, which is now established as safe, acts favorably on all other hormones, except on cortisol, which declines. DHEA and growth hormone also lower cortisol. This is to be taken into account in patients who have low cortisol levels and will require an adjustment to it before taking HGH. Pregnenolone, as a precursor, will naturally increase DHEA levels, which will have to be adjusted downward if this hormone is prescribed.

Progesterone is well known for its anti-estrogen effects, but much less for its anti DHT (dihydrotestosterone) properties. Dr. John R. Lee has highlighted this valuable property of progesterone, and there are now bio-identical progesterone creams for treating benign prostatic hypertrophy or even androgenetic alopecia (25).

There are dozens of hormones in the human body, forty of which are important. Fortunately, I do not encourage you to take them all! The purpose of anti-aging medicine is to detect the deficiencies in the main hormones, and to optimize their rate by a supplementation which must remain **a fraction of the quantity synthesized by the organism, that's the first condition**. Thus, the gland is relieved, the body functions better, and the negative feedback at the hypothalamic pituitary axis is reduced.

The second condition is to use bio-identical hormones and not synthetic molecules. This is essential because the synthetic molecules, whose formula differs, are often more effective but the body does not recognize them and the side effects are often more common and serious.

It is for this reason that HRT (hormone replacement therapy for menopause) has been badly pressured in recent years because prescribed hormones were not bio-identical. For example, estrogen extracted from mare urine or medroxyprogesterone, a toxic synthetic form of natural progesterone has been prescribed. This culminated 15 years ago in a study whose results put forward the potentially carcinogenic side of HRT in menopausal women. Since then, the most recent studies, based on the use of bio-identical estrogen's and progesterone, have all given favorable results on cardiovascular health and the prevention of osteoporosis; so much so that some authors today speak of a "sacrificed generation" for women who have not benefitted from these treatments.

THE THYROIDAL HORMONES, CONDUCTOR OF THE ORCHESTRA

The control of our basal metabolism is essentially exerted by our thyroid hormones. Thyroid hormone deficiency increases with age, in both men and women, even in the absence of autoimmune pathology such as Hashimoto or Basedow. Unfortunately, laboratory blood tests are often bad markers of chronic benign hypothyroidism. Indeed, they give a hormonal image at a time T, which can hide a deficiency that only the dosage of thyroid hormones in the urine from the past 24 hours can highlight (17).

Then there is the problem of TSH laboratory standards (often the only marker used).

According to the medical encyclopedia "Health Medicine", the normal values of TSH are between 0.15 and 5.0 mlU/l.

Yes, you read that right! There is a factor of 30 between the two values!

This means that a patient with a TSH score of 0.15 and another patient with a result of 5.0 will both return home while the second patient has 30 times less TSH than the first. It's like saying that   baking a cake should be between 30°C and 900°C, or that the weight of a normal person is between 30 and 400 kg.

Yet, this is still the reality in 2018.

Hormone treatments are not suitable for the mass treatment protocols of conventional medicine, and the thyroid is probably the most sensitive example. The latest recommendations of the   National Authority for Health continue to consider the TSH as a reliable marker and the T4, inactive hormone, as the treatment of choice for hypothyroidism. Above all, they ignore the major role of cofactors, such as cortisol, vitamin D, selenium, without which the best-fitting treatment will not work well. Finally, one cannot insist enough on a clinical examination which is fundamental in treating thyroid problems.

In fact, for TSH, any result outside the range 0.5-2.5 mlU/l is suspect, the national average being around 1.5 mlU/l. (19)

There is currently a debate about the "health" values of TSH, but this debate is of little importance to me; the TSH being a poor marker of hypothyroidism. Indeed, the determination of the TSH in the blood gives a snapshot, at the moment T of the blood test, of the thyroid function, or more precisely of the hypothalami-pituitary "feedback", the TSH essentially being secreted in front of a T4 deficiency. This value of TSH varies according to the day. Also, although not often prescribed, an assay of T3 and T4 hormones in a 24-hour urine sample will give a much more reliable reflection of thyroid function. Unfortunately, these assays are not routinely performed by all the laboratories, and will be subcontracted to a specialized laboratory.

One cannot stress enough on this point: it is the clinical examination that matters. The signs are numerous and must be alerted. Here are the main ones:

- I struggle getting up in the morning.
- I am cold all the time, particularly the extremities.
- I have dry skin.
- I put on weight easily.

- My face is puffy in the morning.
- I feel like I'm living in slow motion.
- I am often constipated.
- I feel better at the end of the day, particularly when I move about.
- The outer part of my eyebrows are balding (sign of Hertoghe).
- The soles of my feet are often orange.
- I have muscle cramps at night, especially in the calves.
- I have pain in my extremities.
- I have dysbiosis, gastroesophageal reflux.
- I'm depressed.
- I have dry, straw-like hair.

(source: T.Hertoghe Clinic, B. Claeys, S. Résimont)

Treatment is justified when 2 or 3 of these symptoms are observed.

But, is there a simple and easy way to evaluate your thyroid at home?

YES!

One of the best tests is to take your temperature under the tongue (it is the best irrigated area), in the morning once you wake up.

It MUST be, according to researcher Walter Pierpaoli, 36.2 or 36.3 or 36.4. Below these values, hypothyroidism will be suspected; beyond, hyperthyroidism.

Often, when hypothyroidism is detected, it is usually poorly treated. Indeed, the official protocol as taught at the Faculty of Medicine and advised by the **National Authority of Health** in France is to monitor TSH and treat the hormone T4, or thyroxine, who's specialty is best known in France as Levothyrox®. I will not go back to the scandal of Levothyrox® related to its change of excipient. Let's just say that the prescription of Levothryox is the protocol of mass treatment of hypothyroidism.

Alas, this type of treatment can work perfectly for antibiotics, or vitamin D, but not for hormones, including birth control pills, by the way.

Because often, with age, the conversion of the hormone T4 into T3 by the liver (active form) becomes increasingly worse and the patient always feels tired, in spite of a balance of T4 and TSH with the normal values. Other values such as toxic and heavy metals prevent this conversion of the hormone T4 into T3.

In this case, only a treatment associating T3 and T4 will be able to solve the problem.

This treatment exists in the form Euthyral® in France (mixture T3 and T4) or Cynomel® (T3 only) associated in this case with Levothyrox®. The half-life of T4 being much longer than that of T3 (7 days against 24h for T3), this may explain the reluctance of doctors to prescribe the T3- while forgetting Levothyrox® intake has little impact because of its long half life.

Besides these synthetic hormones (however perfectly bio-identical), there are animal thyroid extracts, alas banned in France (Erfa, Armor Thyroid). According to anti-aging physicians, this is the "Rolls" of thyroid supplementation. Indeed, the thyroid extracts have the advantage of containing the whole range of thyroid hormones, T0, T1, T2, T3 and T4, all in a protein matrix that modulates their release into the blood during the day. Some people will look for these extracts in other countries, in Europe or the U.S.A. and swear by this treatment.

However, a well-dosed treatment with synthetic hormones T3 and T4 can bring great benefits (this is the one I've been taking for 20 years), subject to certain reservations, that I will touch further on here.
Imagine that you have successfully balanced your thyroid hormone levels, thanks to the kindness of your endocrinologist, who is very attentive to your complaints and your clinical condition. You have already been lucky, and the work of the practitioner will usually stop here.

But this is not enough...

... it is still necessary that hormones enter the cell!

And yes, this is what I call "functional" hypothyroidism, because, as we will see, the function of hormones is only exercised from the moment they enter the cell. For this, certain elements must be in sufficient quantity in the body. First and foremost, vitamin D (still!), vitamin B12, zinc, cortisol, and selenium. All of these cofactors should be measured in the laboratory because their deficiency may explain a therapeutic failure, despite a normal thyroid status.

A common cause of failure is sometimes failure to treat adrenal insufficiency with cortisol. Again, as for the thyroid, the diagnosis is mostly clinical, blood cortisol dosing being useless, except for rare pathologies like Addison disease.

The thyroid is undoubtedly one of the most fragile glands of the human body. The endocrine disrupters: bromine, fluoride, heavy metals, phthalates and triclosan surround it on all sides do not make it easy. Nor does the growing micronutrient deficit of our modern diet. The impact of the thyroid on the entire body is such that poorly treated deficiency will impact other glands, especially the adrenal glands, which produce cortisol and DHEA. Also, it is recommended to dose these hormones because deficits are common in hypothyroid patients (18).

If we look at the "cascade" of steroid hormones, synthesized from the essential cholesterol, we see that at the top of the chain is pregnenolone. When the adrenal glands are weakened, and when one is under stress, most of the pregnenolone will be used to produce cortisol, to the detriment of other hormones. This is what is called "pregnenolone steal"; and that's why I recommend supplementation (at the dosage of 50mg) from the age of 40 in patients treated for thyroid.

Adrenal function should be evaluated by biological tests AND a thorough clinical examination. See the chapter on cortisol below.

In reality, TSH has a **low diagnostic value.**

And yet we continue to rely on this assay to assess thyroid function.

The causes of hypothyroidism have changed. Formerly, it was mostly related to the lack of iodine. Today, it is mostly a lack of conversion of T4 to T3, and **many sufferers of hypothyroidism have normal test results.**

The fact of associating the dosage of T4 with that of TSH, as I see it every day in the prescriptions of our practitioners, is nonsense, a redundancy, because the first reacts according to the second; and it is much more judicious to measure the T3, whose health values must be in the high statistical values.

I remind you that laboratory norms are statistical values based on an aging population; to ignore it is a serious mistake.

The Euthyral® supplementation will be done **gradually**, by adding a quarter of a tablet, and it may be wise to take a small fraction at noon, because the half life of the T3 is quite short.

Treatment with thyroid hormones is for smart people: it is necessary to identify the clinical signs of hypothyroidism to adjust it regularly; because we generally have a higher need in winter, and decreased in summer.

It has now been established that conventional treatment with Levothyrox (T4) works in about 10 percent of cases, but it may be years before formal recommendations change. Worse, treatments with T4 alone (Levothryox®, Thyroxine®, Thyrofix®) sometimes induce the production of reverse T3 by the body. Reverse T3 is a biologically inactive metabolite associated with increased mortality in the elderly.

To conclude, I will say that the diagnosis of hypothyroidism is done by clinical examination and not by TSH, and that the treatments which work are associated with T4 and T3. Treatment with T4 alone normalizes biology, but not the clinical examination and the patient will often still feel tired after leaving the surgery. Physicians qualified in functional and nutritional medicine are still few in France, but I must mention Dr. Laurent Fogel in Paris, Didier Cosserat in St Raphaël who know and recommend treatments combining T3 and T4.

In the meantime, patients who do not self-educate may suffer longer than they need to.

THE PRODUCTION OF STEROID HORMONES FROM CHOLESTEROL

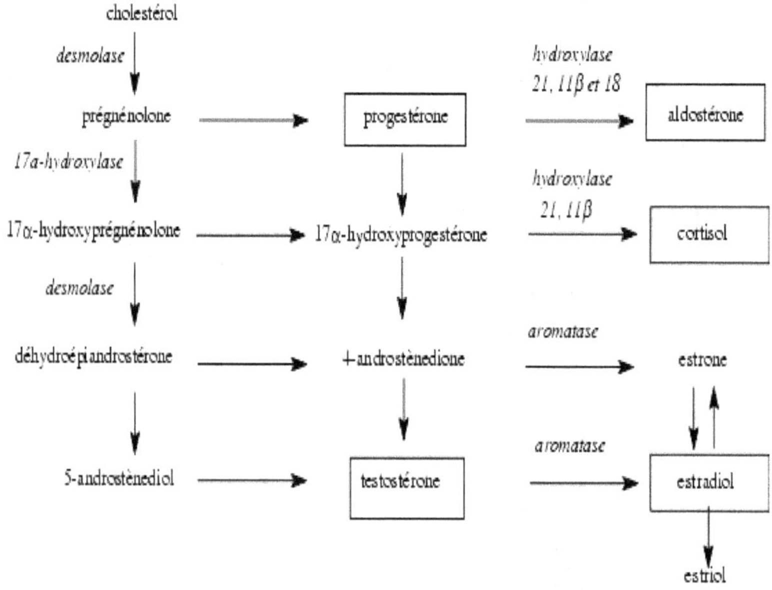

THE MEMORY HORMONE: PREGNENOLONE

Pregnenolone is synthesized directly from cholesterol. It is the "mother" of steroid hormones. It turns the body into a host of other hormones, progesterone, cortisol, D.H.E.A., testosterone, estradiol and aldosterone. This is why a good level of pregnenolone is essential to the hormonal balance. Like many other hormones, it decreases with age.

It is known to play a fundamental role in short-term memorization, but it is a reductive vision to consider it as simply "the memory hormone". I personally see it as the hormonal balance hormone. However, its memory benefits are notable, but take a long time to appear (24). Supplementation can be considered in the forties, when the first "losses" of memory can emerge. This hormone seems very safe, at least as much as the cholesterol it comes from, as long as it is not oxidized.

Pregnenolone helps to solve anxiety problems (20,21). In the U.S.A., where it is over-the-counter, many patients going through hormone therapy have confirmed its positive effects on anxiety.

But, it also helps for attention deficits and even rheumatic pains (at high doses) (22,23).

What laboratory test?

The most valuable laboratory test is Pregnenolone Sulfate. It is important here not to confuse the laboratory standards, which frame 95% of a given population, with the health standards as advocated by the anti-aging medicine.

Thus, the reference values are 40-120 ng/ml, but the optimal values are 90-100 ng/ml. According to some practitioners, this dosage has little effect, BUT pregnenolone supplementation improves the patients' condition and so they continue to be prescribed.

Which dosage to take?

It seems that pregnenolone is still very safe, at least up to 100mg per day. For my part, I supplemented at 50 mg/day for years.

Be careful, taking pregnenolone will probably lead you to reduce your dosage of D.H.E.A., which is logical, the first being the precursor of the second.

The other memory hormone is vasopressin. It is sometimes prescribed in anti-aging medicine, for its property to fight against lines and wrinkles in patients who are deficient. It's finally a more natural alternative to 'botox' - or botulinum toxin - which is highly toxic to the nervous system.

DHEA: ELEXIR OF YOUTH?

DHEA had its glory days in the 90s, thanks to the DHEAge study by Professor Etienne Emile Beaulieu (progesterone world specialist) that made it popular in France.

It is the most powerful anti-aging hormone with growth hormone. It is energizing, so take it in the morning.

Discovered as early as the 1930s, this hormone is at the top of the genesis of steroid hormones just after pregnenolone. It then breaks down into estrogen, androstenediol, testosterone and corticosterone. Long regarded as an elixir of youth, it seems today a little forgotten, probably because its effects are more discreet than other hormones, such as testosterone, or cortisol for example (the latter is widely used in allopathic medicine for its powerful anti-inflammatory properties, alas in the form of the synthetic form of prednisolone (Solupred®), 5 times more potent than the bio-identical form (hydrocortisone) and riddled with side effects when not associated with DHEA to counteract its catabolizing effects.

Yet, DHEA is the most important hormone in the blood (as DHEA sulphate) and it is also one of those that drops most rapidly with age, with melatonin and growth hormone (see the graph of the DHEA above). At sixty, we only have one fifth to one tenth of the rates we had in adolescence. In the last year of life, rates are close to zero. Older women in the Okinawa archipelago in Japan (a "blue zone", known to have a large number of fully independent centenarians) have higher rates of DHEA and testosterone than 75-year-old Western women . Mainly secreted by the adrenals, it plays a key role (but little known) as a moderator of the catabolic effects of cortisol. Besides, that's what to look for: the ratio DHEA / cortisol. In adolescence, it is clearly in favor of DHEA (about 10 times more DHEA than cortisol). And when stress occurs in adolescence, the secretion of cortisol is always accompanied by an increase in DHEA. But with age, cortisol tends to rise (and be less effective, because of the increase in transcortin protein, which limits its free form in the blood) and the DHEA drops so quickly that at age 60 the ratio is almost 1/1. This is one of the reasons why you can not bear stress with age.

The study of Professor Beaulieu has shown its benefits, especially in women, but its effects in humans though discreet are very real - It would have a significant role against cancer, osteoporosis, immunity, energy. Symptoms among people who are deficient include difficulty climbing stairs, and intolerance to noise and stress in general. As I said above, my blood tests showed a clear disability for my age group, and I have been taking it for several years now. Its degradation in testosterone although real is anecdotal to each man: do not count on it to increase your testosterone blood level !. On the other hand, it is noticeable in women (whose testosterone levels are 20 times lower than in men), so much so that it is not recommended to take it without female sex hormones, to avoid its virilizing effects.

However, it does have some anabolic effects: the DHEA helps to maintain a slim and firm body. DHEA also has a protective effect on the skin. Very sensitive about this, I quickly tested this molecule, and checked this property. In humans, when combined with testosterone and growth hormone (via HGH injections or a powerful MK677 secretagogue to adjust IGF1), the effects on the skin are even greater convincing. Contrary to a tenacious belief, which made me hesitate for a long time to test the growth hormone, the increase of the IGF1 is not accompanied by an amplified growth of tumors, on the contrary, I saw my basal cell carcinomas progressively disappear as IGF1 boosts immunity. If we look at the statistical curves of melanoma, women under 50 are more often affected than men, but after 50, the phenomenon is reversed. Scientists argue that this is due to hair loss in humans that no longer protect from the sun's rays. For my part, I think that the androgenic hormones protect the skin of the man but that in the fifties the phenomenon is reversed by the fall of these hormones in the man and by the increase of the estrogen's - all the more marked when the BMI is high.

I remember taking it temporarily in the 90s in U.S.A., where it was already available over the counter. I immediately noted the energizing effect of DHEA, probably because my rates were not that good in my thirties, although I had not done a blood test at that time.

DHEA slows down osteoporosis and has a strong anti-inflammatory effect on the brain. Patients with Alzheimer's have rates that are 50 percent lower than average. It stimulates immunity (hence its effect on the skin and against cancer, mainly with thyroid hormones and growth hormone) and significantly reduces cardiovascular risk. There is an increase in the HDL fraction of cholesterol and a decrease in the LDL fraction.

Be careful though, if you are "borderline" in cortisol, taking DHEA can reduce its production by about 20%. On the other hand, excessive intake results in an increase in estrogen which is not the desired effect, at least in humans.

The maximum dose in adult women is 25 mg, and 50 mg in men. If you are also taking pregnenolone, the dosage will have to be reduced further. For my part, I take 25 mg of DHEA 6 days out of 7, which adjusts my rate around the frequent values of the age group of about 25 years (I take pregnenolone also). In all cases, it is advisable to keep the same mark for follow-up (or the same pharmacy if you use a compound) and to take regular blood tests (DHEA sulphate).

What are the signs of an overdose?

An overdose of DHEA results in oily, shiny skin with pimples, very easy to spot. It is then necessary to gradually lower the dosage. On the internet, there are the usual dosages of 10.25, 50 and 100 mg (useless); but there is always a way, with a prescription, to ask the pharmacist for a different dosage, who will then perform a magistral preparation.

We often hear about poorly dosed capsules on the internet. For my part, I buy it in jar of 300 capsules of 25 mg of a top brand (Vitacost) and now my blood tests are very good.

TESTOSTERONE: IT ALL STARTED WITH A MONKEY'S TESTICLE

One could say that it is thanks to testosterone (albeit unknowingly) that anti-aging medicine started. In France during the 1920s, a Russian surgeon, Samuel Abramovich Voronoff, also known as Serge Voronoff, had the idea of performing testicular transplants from monkeys to elderly and weakened men, even though testosterone had not yet been discovered (26). Initially, the surgeons took the testicles of death row inmates in order to cater to the demands of his rich clients, but, the demand quickly grew. To meet this demand, he embarked on the xenograft of monkeys testes. Greatly admired and then criticized towards the end of his life, this precursor physician paved the way for the future of anti-aging.

Widely used in the sports industry for doping, testosterone has had bad press but wrongly so, it does not deserve such criticism.

This is due once again to the use of identical non-organic toxic forms of testosterone (oral forms such as dianabol, C17-alkylated, highly toxic to the liver and rightly banned in France) or its derived synthetic forms, commonly known as anabolic steroids that are widely used in doping (Deca durabolin, Primobolan, Anavar, Turinabol etc). These forms of synthesis have been formulated to maximize the anabolic effect of testosterone and minimize the effects of virilization. As for the same non-organic cortisone, the side effects are numerous because the body does not recognize these molecules. In addition, in the very particular context of doping, the doses used exceed by several tens of times the recommended physiological dose!

In reality, in both men and women (at doses 20 times lower in women, however), testosterone plays a vital role in well-being. Coupled with a paleo-style diet, it helps burn fat almost as well as growth hormone. It optimizes the lipid balance as well as improving insulin sensitivity. Women who are deficient often have cellulite. In hypo-gonadal men, we often (not always) notice being overweight, an increase in the thoracic perimeter (typical of andropause), visceral fat, and especially a decrease in motivation and energy, even depression. It also boosts tissue irrigation. A specialist doctor in testosterone, Dr. Muller, a Danish man from Copenhagen, treats diabetic patients with gangrene with high doses of testosterone.

The success of testosterone supplementation is largely related to the nutrition that accompanies it, as I said above. In this case, it can work wonders; to the point that many men under TRT (Testosterone Replacement Therapy) claim they were "zombies" before treatment and that they really noticed a difference after having TRT. The success of the treatment is also due to a fine adjustment of the dosage, and a good management of the natural catabolites of testosterone, estradiol and dihydrotestosterone (DHT). When these conditions are met, which requires a real investment from the patient, the TRT can not only be very beneficial, but long-term.

Above all, the deficiency must be proven by the clinic and laboratory tests. The andropause balance sheet will contain at least the following parameters:

- Blood count
- Total and bioavailable testosterone
- P.S.A
- FSH and LH
- DHEA sulphate
- Estradiol (if possible high-sensitivity technique, unfortunately not available in Europe)

An attempt will be made to establish whether hypogonadism is primary or secondary (due to poor feedback of the hypothalamic pituitary axis or testicular deficiency). The decline of testosterone is normal when one ages (about 1% per year from 30 years) but that is not the same for everyone. What's worse, it seems that in recent years, we encounter more and more hypogonadism in young men, whereas it was rarely seen in the past - except for certain pathologies, for example testicular cancer - to treat someone younger than 45. According to specialists like Dr. Hertoghe, deficits can occur at any age, including newborns.

Endocrine disruptors have some importance. Most are "estrogen-like", that is, they mimic female sex hormones. This results in early puberty in young girls, and sometimes hypogonadism in men. They also act negatively on fertility (which has been know to have effected fish for a long time).

A deleterious way of life does not help things. Thus, the consumption of alcohol, processed meats, cheeses and processes foods have a negative impact on testosterone and promote its aromatization of estrogen, an enzymatic phenomenon that we recall is mainly found in adipose tissue.

Also called muscle hormone, a testosterone deficiency will result in a soft and loose body. Its action on the mind may explain depression during your forties, not responding to classic psychotropic drugs. Its role in anti-aging medicine is obvious: it fight against sarcopenia (age-related muscle wasting), osteoporosis and atherosclerosis by fortifying the heart muscle and the endothelium of the arteries. After 50, testosterone helps prevent metabolic syndrome, visceral fat, and tissue softening in general. It also helps to strengthen the walls of our arteries. It would also be sensible to check the vascular health of the patient before starting the treatment, because testosterone has the property of being able to "remove" the atheromatous plaque.

Which forms of testosterone?
Once clinical hypogonadism has been established, along with an assay (generally starting at 3 ng/ml or below the ideal level being around 7-8 ng/ml in humans) hormonal supplementation should be considered. There are many formulas in the US, from patches to "pellets", to liposomal creams prepared in a "compounding pharmacy" or more conventional injections (the ester used in the US is cypionate). All are bioidentical forms and may be suitable depending on the needs of each patient.

In anti-aging medicine, the 10% liposomal testosterone cream for men is favored by practitioners. It avoids overdose and the use of injections. However, it does have its downfalls: there is a risk of contamination when applied to the skin by contact, and it tends to generate a lot of DHT (dihydrotestosterone) under the effect of the enzyme 5 alpha reductase, present in the skin tissue. On the other hand, liposomal creams are only available in "compounding" pharmacies in magistral preparation and required fairly expensive equipment. One of them, based in Frankfurt, on behalf of "Receptura" can manufacture these creams a prescription basis.

In France, there is an oral form of testosterone, Pantestone®, which is supposed to avoid the first pass through the liver and go through the lymphatic system: in practice, it is often not very effective in the long term.

There is also Androgel®, but its dosage is too low to have a noticeable effect in many cases.

There is also a hydroalcoholic gel, called Andractim®, but I recommend it for the treatment of andropause: it is actually dihydrotestosterone (DHT). Its use can be considered for a local treatment against gynecomastia, due to the anti-estrogen effects of this molecule. However, in the long run, DHT makes the prostate swell and causes hair loss.

Lastly are the injections, in the ester form, the testosterone molecule becomes bioavailable because it breaks down slower. Thus testosterone enanthate has a half-life of about 5 days (Androtardyl®), testosterone undecanoate takes about several weeks allowing a space between injections (Nebido®).

Testosterone enanthate: official protocol versus latest practices in the U.S.A

The official protocol is to administer 250mg of testosterone enanthate intramuscularly every 2 to 4 weeks. However, this generates too many variations: in the first few days, the levels reached are clearly supra physiological (> 10 ng/ml), but as of the second week, they fall very quickly. We then witness a roller coaster that in the end, is not very beneficial for the patient.

The subcutaneous route, a solution?

In recent years, the practice of subcutaneous injection by some TRT practitioners have appeared in the US. Viewed with suspicion, studies in hindsight showed that despite the fact that the product was injected into an area rich in adipose tissue, the conversion of estrogen from testosterone was not greater than the conventional intramuscular route. Better, some practitioners (Dr.Crisler, USA) noted in the patients using this route that a smaller amount of testosterone was needed to achieve the same plasma levels as with the intramuscular route.

Today, more and more patents prefer to split injections (1 or 2 per week); injections that can actually be done subcutaneously in a much more comfortable way. This is the protocol currently used in the USA.

Testosterone: frequent values

Laboratory norms are 2.5 to 10 ng/ml.

The optimal rates recommended in anti-aging medicine are between 6 and 8 ng/ml - depending on the size of the patient.

Side effects and parameters to look for.

1. Hematocrits

The percentage of red blood cells in the blood is increased because the cells are boosted by testosterone. This explains the anaemia and pale complexion in men who lack it. If the hematocrits rise above the frequent values (quite rare), then blood donation is required.

2. P.S.A

PSA or Prostate Specific Antigen is a marker of prostatic activity. Although recent studies have failed to demonstrate that testosterone has an initiating role in prostate cancer, it is common to monitor the evolution of this marker after the age of 50 in France. It is interesting to note that this surveillance by the PSA has been abandoned in the USA.

The fact that prostate adenoma problems develop in elderly men seems to confirm the rather protective role of testosterone with respect to the prostate. This is what emerges in any case from the most recent studies on the subject. Estrogen's and dihydrotestosterone (DHT) would have a rather detrimental influence on the prostate over time.

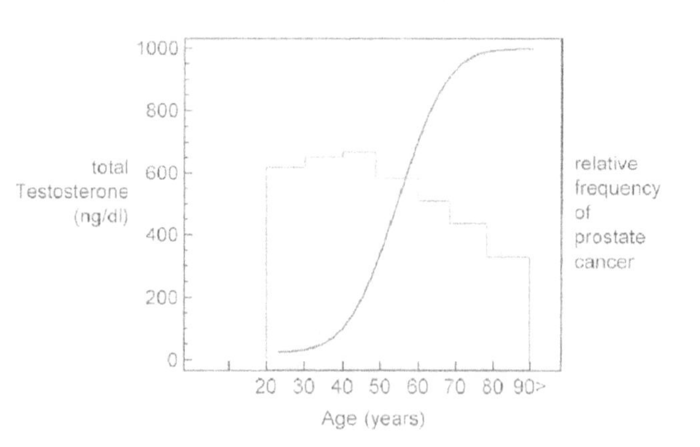

3. Arterial tension: an urban legend

No, testosterone therapy does not increase blood pressure. On the contrary, by strengthening the arteries, it influences the evolution of the arteries during aging.

4. Controlling estrogen

As we have seen for DHEA, an excess of testosterone can result in an increase in estrogen beyond reason. It is therefore important to limit testosterone intake to what is strictly necessary, and to control the level of estradiol (E2) regularly. Some plants such as chrysin are known and sometimes used to limit aromatization. Foods such as coffee, sugar and cold cuts, cheeses and alcohol also favor the rise of estrogen. If the E2 is too high, an aromatase inhibitor such as anastrozole (Arimidex®) may be used in a very small amount over a short period of time. The use of this anti-aromatase is "off-label" and should be limited over time, if possible. Indeed, the latest studies have shown a risk of osteoporosis during prolonged use of these products. A DEXA examination is then recommended to evaluate this decalcification.

GROWTH HORMONE : THE "RULER" HORMONE.

The rate of HGH, or Human Growth Hormone, drops very rapidly with age (see graph below measuring the level of IGF1 vs. age). Curve 95 corresponds to 95 percentile: this means that only 5% of the population is above this curve - same as curve 5 for low values. We can see a sharp drop in the IGF1 level before the age of 30, then a stabilization, and a net recovery from the fall towards age 60.

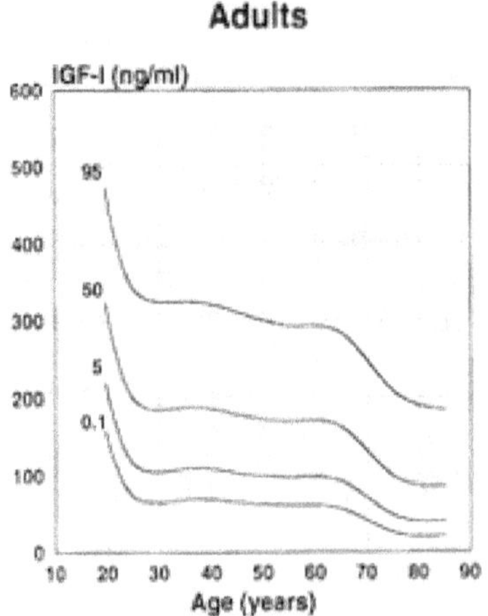

For many doctors, this hormone is only for the growth of children. This is almost the only indication in France to treat children with severe growth delays. Yet, its effects on the health of adults go well beyond that and are attested by many studies. To tell the truth, few molecules with so-called "anti-aging" properties managed to pass the

96

double-blind, placebo-controlled trial, the "gold standard" in this area.

HGH has passed this test brilliantly, many times even.

On July 5th, 1990, the prestigious *New England Journal of Medicine* published the results of a study of men aged 61 to 81 who had shock wave treatment. While the control continued to age normally, the effects on the synthetic HGH-treated group (naturally produced by the pituitary gland) were described by Dr. Daniel Rudman, MD, in these terms: "The effects of 6 months HGH on lean body mass and adipose-tissue mass were equivalent in magnitude to the changes incurred during 10 to 20 years of aging." (28).

The grey hair of a 65-year-old man became brown again. The woman of another volunteer in the study, although younger by 15 years, had trouble managing her husband's increased energy. A third saw the wrinkles on his face start to fade.

Today, this type of result is experienced every day for the lucky ones who can be treated in anti-aging clinics in the USA, or in that of Dr. Hertoghe in Brussels; but unfortunately not in France, where the use of HGH for anti-aging purposes is prohibited.

It must be said that things started badly in France. For a long time, a delay in children's growth was treated with HGH taken from the pituitary glands of dead bodies, even though other countries were already synthesizing it by bacterial recombinant DNA (a manufacturing process similar to that of insulin) much safer from a health point of view. Thus, the scandal of Kreutzfeld Jacob's disease broke out when patients started to suffer from prion diseases.

Yet, the list of beneficial effects of HGH is growing as studies progress, here are a few examples out of many:

- 8.8% muscle growth in 6 months without exercise
- 14.4% average fat loss after 6 months without special diets
- increase in energy
- Improved libido
- Growth of the heart, liver, kidneys and all organs that shrink with age
- Healing and accelerated healing
- Improved immunity
- Insomnia in old men is restored with deep sleep
- Lowered blood pressure
- Improved vision
- Boost in hair growth
- Increased memory
- Wrinkles fade
- Improved lipid profile
- Reinforced bone structure
- Increase sports performance

Most of these effects are attributable to the increase in IGF1 synthesized by the liver at the instigation of HGH (Insulin-Like Growth Factor 1) but not only.

It is also called "the ruler hormone" because it provides a state of serenity and calm, and allows multitasking without feeling any stress.

Conversely, the patient deficient in growth hormone will complain of immense fatigue, impossible to diminish. Skin becomes saggier, especially above the knees and deep wrinkles appear more visible on the face, and the back tends to bend.

How can one control their growth hormone levels?

Almost undetectable in the blood, it is necessary to measure the level of IGF1 to evaluate its secretion. Some authors also recommend that the transport protein, IGFBP3 - the equivalent of SHBG for for testosterone, be assayed to evaluate the free form of IGF1.

How to improve secretion naturally?
It is secreted at night mainly but there may be peaks in the day, driven in particular by a sports activity, but not just any. Indeed, it is the high-intensity fractional exercise that is most effective for triggering an HGH peak. Namely: lift weights in sets (squats, press, deadlift, bench press, in the form of intense sets, or short sprints with short rest periods etc.)

Cardio marathon sessions or pool lengths are therefore not ideal because any exercise exceeding the duration of 45 minutes to 1 hour triggers the secretion of catecholamines and cortisol, aka catabolic stress hormones.

There are secretagogues, ie products that stimulate the secretion of HGH.

Arginine or Ornithine has been talked about for a long time, but it turns out that it takes high doses of several grams to have an effect. Low-dose glutamine (2g) seems to be more effective in the elderly. I rather recommend the amino acid glycine, which mixed with an infusion for example, can substitute sugar for it sweet flavor. In addition to boosting HGH, glycine is also a precursor or collagen and glutathione. Finally, there are other secretagogues that do not have Marketing

Authorization (MA), such as ipamorelin (in injection form) or MK677 (ghrelin analogue, taken orally). However, they have shown their effectiveness in increasing IGF1 without effecting the response to cortisol.

It is also important to be careful of the "miracle products" on the internet - starting with oral HGH (this is impossible, HGH is a fragile peptide made up of 191 amino acids and cannot be taken this way) or "Pseudo HGH" homeopathic. Anyway, if you want to test the effectiveness of these products, only a dosage of IGF1 before and 6 weeks after can confirm the effectiveness of the treatment.

The hormones that most influence the secretion of HGH are T3, testosterone and estradiol.

Growth Hormone Treatment

It is difficult to obtain a quality growth hormone in France for anti-aging purposes. In addition to Western pharmaceutical brands (Norditropin®, Humatrope®, Saizen® etc...), there are Chinese manufacturers (Jintropin®, Godtropin®...). Not all of them are necessarily bad, especially when they come with an analysis certificate, but they will have to be tested in the laboratory.

In all cases, administration is subcutaneous. Western brands often offer the pen form, like for insulin, which makes accurate dosing and injection easy. For other forms, you will find bacteriostatic water for injections, not found in France. Only this water, which contains a low dose of benzyl alcohol, will keep in a reconstituted flask for 15 days, this peptide being very fragile as soon as it is reconstituted.

It should begin with low doses, less than 1 IU, and monitor the evolution of IGF1 over the months. It is a treatment that should last at least 3 to 4 months. There is no reported negative pituitary feedback; it would even seem that, as for melatonin, the treatment often "wakes up" the gland and that smaller doses are needed over time.

My experience:

After 6 weeks, an excessive dosage of HGH had raised my IGF1 to 400 ng/ml (ideal rate around 250 ng/ml depending on the reagent kits and technique used). I spent my time sleeping and eating, and I lowered the doses. I have never had carpal tunnel syndrome, reported side effect in those who take too high doses. Also, take care here to monitor cortisol and thyroid activity.

The effects on the skin ("baby skin") appear quickly over the weeks. This is with high-quality sleep (it makes dreams very "colorful", hyperrealistic), the most reported effect in patients.

Skeptical about the effectiveness of commercially available secretagogues, I decided to test one, the MK677, a mimetic of ghrelin (the appetite hormone) to see it it proved more effective than ipamorelin - already tested with a mean result on IGF1. My protocol was a single dose at bedtime of 20mg of oral MK677 (ibatumoren) combined with 3mg of melatonin MZS - one of the best forms of melatonin on the market, developed by Dr. Pierpaoli.

After only five weeks, the results were clear: while ipamorelin had given IGF1 at 220 ng/ml, the MK677 increased the rate up to 330 ng/ml, a value too high for anti-aging therapy! I was starting to suffer from joint paint and I had to stop the treatment after 5 weeks. I have decided to test a lower dosage of 10mg of MK677 at a later date.

This experiment has made it possible to demonstrate that, contrary to what some authors think, it is still possible to stimulate the production of HGH by the pituitary, even beyond the age of 50.

What about acromegaly?

Acromegaly is a rare disease induced by a tumor (often benign) of the pituitary gland that causes an almost permanent secretion of HGH. It is often found in those in their forties, belatedly detected, it causes progressive deformation of the face and extremities, accompanied by severe fatigue. When it comes to adolescence and growth is not achieved, we talk about gigantism. Excess growth hormone can cause diabetes as part of acromegaly; but it must be remembered that the rates are very excessive and have nothing to do with the dosages of anti-aging medicine. Contrary to belief, acromegalic sufferers are less affected than the general population for all cancers combined, except colon cancer.

Richard Kiel ("Shark" in James Bond) or "André the Giant" are famous acromegaly sufferers in Hollywood cinema.

CORTISOL : THE TWO-FACED HORMONE

In general opinion, cortisone is a treatment of last resort, to avoid as far as possible as there are numerous side effects such as osteoporosis, diabetes, hypertension, water retention etc. In fact, cortisol is so essential to the human body that a defect causes death within 24 hours. The dramatic side effects chart that I have just outlined are largely due to the use of identical non-organic synthetic corticoids such as prednisolone to name only the best known (Solupred®). These synthetic forms are 5 times more powerful than hydrocortisone (the identical bio molecule used in anti-aging medicine). In addition, doctors prescribe it in massive doses (1mg/kg in general) that prohibit its use over time.

According to Dr. Hertoghe, 30 to 40 percent of adults have cortisol deficiency which starts between 20-30 years of age. Recall that according to laboratory standards, only 2.5 percent of the population is deficient in cortisol.

The most common signs are a hollowed face, dark circles under the eyes, pigmented spots on the face, conjunctivitis (sign of poorly controlled chronic inflammation), allergies, low blood pressure, clammy hands due to compensation of catecholamines under stress.

In addition to clinical examination, the most sensitive laboratory tests to detect deficiency are 24-hour urine testing or a transcortin blood test (also called CBG, for Cortisol Binding Globulin). For my part, it is the transcortin and the clinical examination that alerted me. A high level of of transcortin signifies a cortisol deficiency.

There is also an ACTH test, but this one seems controversial because the ACTH levels commonly used are too high and even worsen the adrenal glands.
A supplementation of only 10mg per day of hydrocortisone in the morning, combined with an infusion of Perilla Frutescens (see the chapter on alopecia for the description of this plant) was enough to solve my allergy problem, lowered tension and the frequent use of antihistamines. This treatment also stopped the sugar craving I would often get in the afternoon.

It is estimated that the average man secretes 22.5mg per day of cortisol, and women 9.2mg (depending on body surface area). Thus, a supplementation of 10 or 15mg represents only a fraction of this secretion and induces little or no negative feedback on the adrenal glands. One must take care to take the maximum when waking up and the last taken at noon to respect the natural cycle of cortisol, whose rates are naturally high in the morning and low in the late afternoon. As I have already written above, you must always counterbalance a cortisol intake with DHEA.

Taken in excess, cortisol will cause bruising, a puffy face and water retention.

At the recommended dosage by anti-aging medicine, cortisol helps to burn fat, reduces fatigue and helps to cope with stress (29).

In reality, the adipose tissue often seen in patients treated with cortisone does not come from the hormone itself, but from its stimulating effect on the appetite - an effect all the stronger as the dose is high and the identical non-organic molecule.

Cortisol even has antioxidant properties, in addition to its well-known anti-inflammatory effects. By neutralizing free radicals, it minimizes tissue damage during stressful situation where high levels of free radicals are produced (30,31,32). That's why I call it "the two-sided hormone". Finally, as I said above, cortisol is essential to get T3 thyroid hormone into the cell. Also any deficiency in cortisol will have an impact on the thyroid activity.

How to increase the secretion of cortisol naturally?
1. Sun exposure.
Every time you are exposed to the sun, secretion increases by 5 percent in a few minutes.

2. Take Vitamin C
By boosting the surrenals, Vitamin C will increase cortisol secretion.

3. Avoid high-sugar intake.
Cortisol deficiency often induces sweet craving at the end of day, which in turn lower the secretion cortisol. A vicious circle to avoid.

4.Take licorice root extract, ashwaganda or certain plants.
Licorice is known to mimic the effects of cortisol and can relieve people who lack it. There are also plants that can be easily found on the internet , which boost the adrenal (type "adrenal support" on Google).

In any case, a prolonged treatment with hydrocortisone is justified as soon as the deficiency is proved, because the deficient patients suffer a lot (one speaks about "paranoia") and often make those close to them suffer.
After establishing the type of impairment (primary, secondary or tertiary) with the help of the

doctor, treatment can be established - always under medical supervision and with DHEA, whose anabolic effects counterbalance those of cortisol.

MELATONIN AND THE PINEAL GLAND : PROVEN IMPACT ON LONGEVITY.

In the general opinion, melatonin is just a product used by frequent travelers to help them recover fast from jet lag. It is difficult to find a more reductive definition. The kinetics of melatonin are quite unique. Indeed, like many other hormones it drops with age and the decline begins at puberty. This is explained today by the fact that the pineal gland (which secretes melatonin) is in a way, the biological clock of our body. We are designed to reproduce ourselves, and this drop of secretion from puberty would send a signal to our body to start aging.
Basically, this means that, from an evolutionary point of view, we do not serve much of the purpose for our group after reproduction. Indeed, it has been observed that the pineal gland often calcifies with age, inevitably slowing down its secretory activity (melatonin and TRH, but also certain other peptides, discovered later). Melatonin is an almost ubiquitous hormone: it is found everywhere, including in the plant kingdom.
It is not yet produced on your first days of life, but it is found in breast milk. Some experts explain the excitement of bottle-fed babies born with a lack of melatonin during the first days of life. The pineal gland is really our body clock: it secretes other hormones, such as TRH (which stimulates, among other things, the secretion of TSH, which, in turn, activates the thyroid), and another peptide, epitalon (formerly called epithalamine). This

peptide was isolated by the late Vladimir Dilman of the N.N. Petrov Research Institute of Oncology of St. Petersburg, Russia. Experiments on rats have shown, like melatonin, that epitalon increases longevity and slows down aging.

Dr. Pierpaoli has demonstrated in multiple mouse studies the effect of melatonin on longevity (13). In a first experiment, he gave a group of NZB (New Zealand Black) mice water supplemented with melatonin, the control group having just received tap water. The normal lifespan of a laboratory mouse is around 24 months. This is what was observed in the control group: they all died after 24 months, often with cancerous lesions. In contrast, the treated group lived 4 to 6 months longer, and the autopsy did not reveal any cancerous lesions just a classical age-related organ atrophy.
The exact figures of the study are 715 days on average for the control group versus 843 days for the treated mice. No visible effects were detected during diurnal administration of melatonin, and no difference in weight between the two groups.

This increase of longevity corresponds, if extrapolated to humans, to 25 years of additional life in good health. Above all, the treated mice had a thymus larger than mice, aged less quickly, and seemed to resist diseases more easily.

To go further, he transplanted pineal glands of aged mice into young mice (thanks to the know-how equipment of the "stereotaxic" surgical procedures developed by his Russian colleagues): the mice have aged faster than normal. The reverse was also true: the young-on-old transplant extended the life of the group. Dr Pierpaoli concludes: "Whatever the mechanism, the transplantation of young pineal results in the preservation of the immune response, and a morphological restoration of the thymus and thyroid occurs at a time when the normal involution of the age is observable. Our exogenous use of circadian melatonin and young pineal gland grafts at the thymus site in older mice suggests that there may be a real relationship between the pineal, its products and the thymus, which provides a mechanism Homeostatic control of size for aging and survival.

It was, however, from a technical point of view, far from being a celebrated case: if the pineal gland of a human is the size of a pea that of a mouse is the size of a full stop.

A major antioxidant

Melatonin is not a simple antioxidant, like vitamin C for example. It is both water-soluble and fat-soluble, which gives it the property of acting in all the compartments of the body. Studies have shown that it has a strong affinity for the nucleus of cells, and that it "repairs" them during the night. At the Third Conference on Cancer and Ageing in Stromboli, Dr.Russel Reiter made a presentation entitled "Melatonin as a Free-radical Scavenger: Implications for Ageing and Age-related Disease". Its role inside the nucleus, confirmed in cell culture, is to protect the DNA but, this anti-oxidant property should not overshadow its major role as a conductor.

The conductor of other hormones

Melatonin sends messages to all other glands. This is a message that the body is young and needs to optimize its hormones. By secreting TRH, the pineal gland activates the thyroid. With age, the decline in TRH inevitably affects thyroid activity. By modulating the enzyme deiodinase, melatonin facilitates the transformation of the hormone T4 (inactive) into hormone T3 (active). This transformation is getting worse and worse today, under the harmful influence of heavy metals, endocrine disruptors. This is why there are so many clinical signs of hypothyroidism in people with normal biological balance but I have already developed this topic in the chapter on thyroid. Melatonin activates the secretion of growth hormone during the night and lowers that of cortisol, the excess of which can be harmful to the tissues.

Development of the thymus and maintaining immunity

The thymus is an organ that declines rapidly with age, and is replaced with a fatty mass. Melatonin-treated mice lived longer than control mice largely because they survived age-related diseases such as autoimmune diseases and cancer. Many studies show the ability of melatonin to inhibit the development of cancer cells. It has been shown to improve the effectiveness of chemotherapy. That's why chemotherapy is better supported when given at night. Today, we study the anti-cancer properties of melatonin at very high doses (over 100mg). All mice treated with melatonin maintained their volume of thymus over time, unlike untreated mice. Dr. Pierpaoli's book is not new, it goes back to the 1990s. Yet, it seems that the government has not retained its encouraging message on immunity, while the incidence of cancer continues to rise over the years. Regarding other infectious agents, the scope of vaccination, with the new "vaccine cocktails" appears more and more insufficient, at a time when viruses are more numerous with a high capacity for mutation across the globe. The melatonin track, like that of vitamin D, should be studied more seriously. It is all the more interesting because acts on diseases before it is too late. Unfortunately, these two natural molecules are not patentable: that probably explains the lack of interest of pharmaceutical industry to launch studies on the subject.

Promising effects on ocular pathologies such as D.M.L.A

Macular degeneration is typically a disease related to aging, like cataracts. A recent study of about 100 patients with AMD (both forms, "wet and dry") showed a visible improvement in Ophthalmological examination within 6 months after treatment with melatonin at the conventional dose of 3mg per os. This improvement continued until the 24th month, marking the end of the study. The results are very encouraging and need to be confirmed by other studies. In a way, they confirm the personal experience of Dr.Hertoghe, who had noticed an improvement in his eyesight when he was given epitalon, another peptide secreted by the pineal gland.

What form of melatonin: sublingual, oral, and at what dosage?

Melatonin is hard to absorb orally. Sublingually, 0.5 to 1mg maximum is sufficient. It must be taken 3 more times orally.

According to Pierpaoli, it should not be taken before age 45 with the following dosages:

45-54 years ...... 1 to 2mg at bedtime
55-64 years ...... 2 to 2.5mg at bedtime
65-74 years ...... 2.5 to 5mg at bedtime
75 years and over ...... 3.5 to 5mg at bedtime

Dosages seem to vary significantly from one individual to another. It is advisable to proceed in steps of 0.5mg, and to lower the dose if it is difficult to wake up the next morning. Many anti-aging physicians or specialists in functional and nutritional medicine prescribe a sublingual form. Having taken it for several years, I can say that it has a major flaw. Falling asleep is fast, but you wake up sometimes in the middle of the night because of the time you took it. In reality, the peak of melatonin should take place around 1am to 2am. Dr Pierpaoli has developed an oral form of melatonin, coupled with two major co-factors (zinc and selenium), with excipients causing its release around 2am, when taken between 22h and 23h. This melatonin, called MZS®, is the one I recommend. You can find it on the vita-stream.com website.

ANDROGENIC ALOPECIA or how to grow back your hair at 50 years old.

Many men are sooner or later confronted with the problem of hair loss. When the phenomenon occurs early, sometimes in your twenties, it can be quite embarrassing. There is even a story in the Old Testament (chapters 13-16): it is that of the Samson warrior, who was endowed with great strength, and could defy an entire army, but he had a weak point. When Dalila had cut his hair, he lost all his strength. Some young men experience alopecia in the same way, and lose confidence in themselves with they self-esteem taking a hit.

There are several types of alopecia, and the treatments may differ. In this chapter, I will only deal with androgenic alopecia, the one that responds to hormonal treatments.

In my case, my family history seemed to have already charted the road. As far back as I can remember, I have always known my father with baldness that has developed over the years, and my paternal grandfather has always been completely bald. Despite this, I was able to keep my hair long enough, at least until my forties - despite a clearing of the temples that is already visible. However, at the dawn of 50 years old, I had at least level 3 alopecia according to the Norwood classification (see below). While evolution had been slow so far, my hair had become very thin and increasingly clear or white and was falling out more frequently over the weeks.

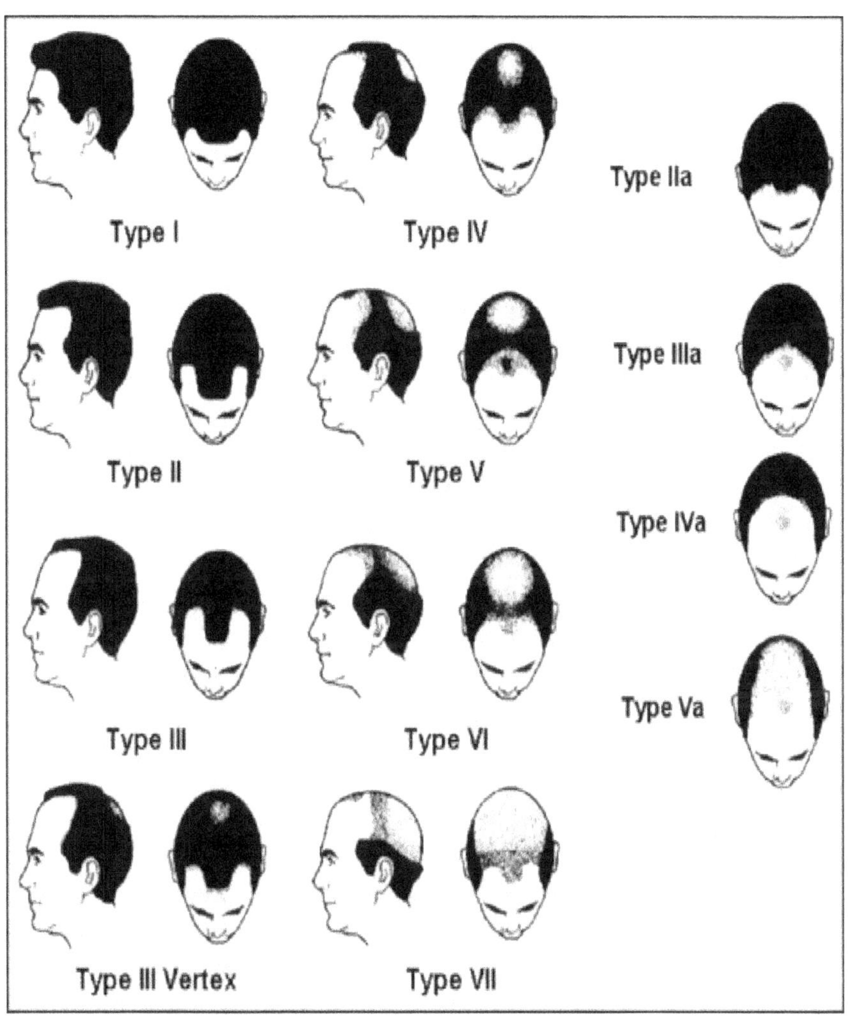

I began to document the existing treatments. I learned that besides the aesthetic aspect, alopecia hides a darker side: there is 2.5 times more prostate cancer in men who have lost their hair at a young age. Worse, those who have significant baldness on the top of the skull are three to four times more likely to have a heart attack! (33,34 and 35). Another concern I have is that, living in the tropics all year round with fair skin and a history of melanoma, it became imperative to lose as little hair as possible.

For me, who was already following an anti-aging treatment for a few years, I could not let this loss progress any longer, especially since I knew that it was synonymous with hormonal and nutritional deficiencies as well as reduced health. Also, I decided on a graft as a last resort. I started with minoxidil at 5% at first. This product, originally designed for blood pressure problems, has proven to be an effective stimulant on follicles. I think I slowed the fall somewhat, applying it religiously twice a day, but after the three years, I had to face the facts: the phenomenon accelerated more and more. I had to either stop or move onto to something more powerful. I knew that androgenic alopecia was largely due to a hormone, dihydrotestosterone (DHT), which is a breakdown product of testosterone, whose levels increase with age under the action of an enzyme, the 5 alpha reductase. Contrary to popular belief, testosterone does not cause hair loss. On the contrary, it makes hair thick and strong. The whole problem comes from the DHT. In addition, high levels of DHT are often accompanied by a hypertrophy of the prostate, a problem that must be avoided at all costs. I had to resolve it by testing an inhibitor of 5 alpha reductase, finasteride. This product is 100% chemical, the reason for hesitating to use it for so long. In addition, the possible side effects reported on the libido limit the use after 45 years and I exceeded the limit. However, these side effects are quite rare and especially occur when the testosterone levels are already low in the patient, which is not my case. I could therefore try the treatment. Fortunately, after several weeks of finasteride, there was no problem with my libido. As with many other chronic conditions however, I knew in my heart that it took a global approach to overcome my alopecia, the failure of minoxidil was there to remind me of it.

That's when I met Alex R., blogger in Oslo, Norway (36). His story is that of an early and sever alopecia (from his twenties) that he managed to completely reverse by acting on four factors. That's what I missed in my protocol. His approach is as follows:

1. Limit the production of DHT (finasteride, ketoconazole shampoo and supplements).
2. Limit inflammation of the scalp with plant extract (Perilla Frutescens)
3. Stimulate follicles with minoxidil. He recommends using a derma roller for the scalp beforehand, which promotes absorption of minoxidil (and activates microcirculation at the same time). One single application per day in the evening is enough.
4. Consume all the necessary nutritional elements that promote healthy hair.

I already knew the famous "Big 3" as the British call it. Basically, it's a combination of finasteride, minoxidil, and a ketoconazole shampoo. This type of protocol works at 80% which is not bad but compared to Alex was not enough to increase chances of success. So, I started Alex's protocol in January 2018, adding injection of biotin and intramuscular Byzantine to boost hair growth. Subsequently, I continued to take biotin, orally. You can use the simplified or complete protocol according to your budget. Here is the treatment in more detail:

Simplified protocol:
1. Finasteride 1.25 mg
2. 2. Minoxidil 5% (Rogaine®) foam after massage of the scalp with a derma roller (1.5mm).
3. Perilla Frutescens (a plant that is widely consumed in Asia, with anti inflammatory and anti-allergic properties). It comes in the form of capsules (Allermin®, Finnish site) or in the form of leaves (Amazon) to be consumed as an infusion.
4. Regenepure® ketoconazole shampoo. This agent (known anti-fungal) has anti DHT properties on the scalp, and anti inflammatory. Use 6 days out of 7, at night, before applying minoxidil. The Revita® shampoo, is of high quality and worth trying, even if it no longer contains ketoconazole in its formulation. Personally, I use both shampoos alternately.

Full protocol:

This is the same as the above, with these dietary supplements:
- Lysine (amplifies the effect of finasteride) 1g
- Taurine (anti DHT) 1g
- Maxi Hair Plus from Country Lab (complete blend with biotin, B vitamins, zinc) 4 capsules
- Nettle leaf (400 mg) anti DHT
- Powdered brewer's yeast, incorporated into diet.

FOCUS ON FINASTERIDE

Finasteride (Propecia®, Chibro Proscar®) acts on one of the two isoenzymes of 5 alpha reductase. It is a derivative of progesterone. The recommended dosage against alopecia is 1mg per day but it has been reported on the forums to have good effects on hair growth from 0.5mg. Some push the dosage up to 2.5mg (See Dr. Hertoghe's program). I strongly advise to do a total testosterone dosage before considering hormonal treatment with finasteride.

Indeed, this molecule can significantly decrease libido and cause atrophy of the genitals in the case of low levels of testosterone not corrected by supplementation. This recommendation is even more important for those over 45 years old. The formulation called Chibro Proscar® is dosed at 5mg because it is intended to treat prostatic hypertrophy. The problem of Propecia (dosed at 1mg) is that it costs 7 times more than Proscar, because it is considered a comfort medicine. A good compressed cut can bypass the problem: it is enough to cut into 4 Proscar tablets.

Dutasteride (Advodart®) is more potent than finasteride because it inhibits both isoenzymes of 5 alpha reductase. The negative effects reported on the libido are more common, that's why I do not recommend it.

NATURAL ALTERNATIVE TO FINASTERIDE

Saw Palmetto extract is known to naturally inhibit the production of DHT and is frequently used against benign prostatic hypertrophy. I have no feedback regarding its use against androgenic alopecia. On the other hand, according to some authors, its negative effects on libido are more frequent than those of finasteride.

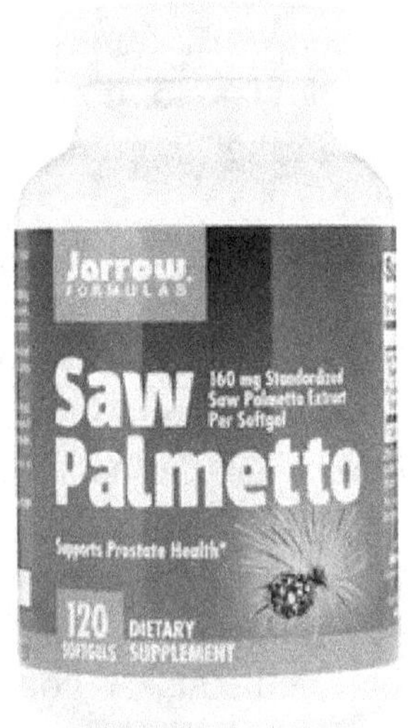

RESULTS

First results (it's my scalp!). At 7 months of treatments (vertex zone):

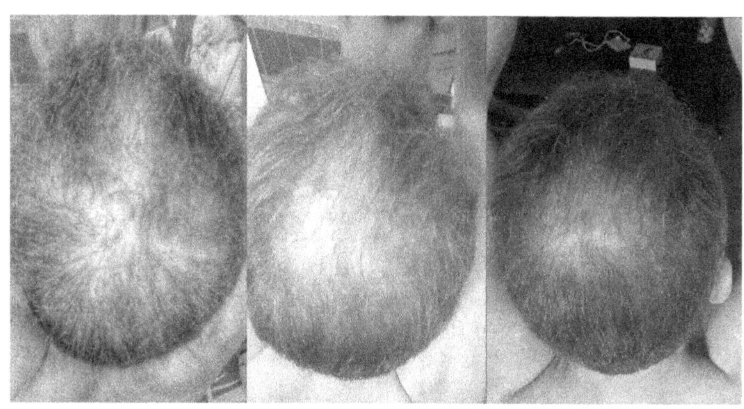

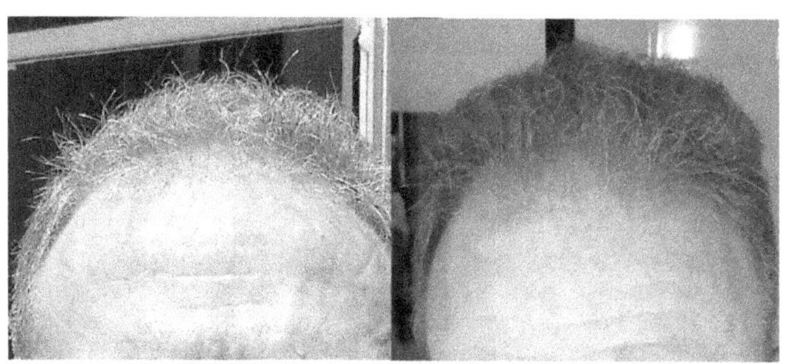

The first effects appear on the frontal area after 3 to 6 months. The results on the vertex appear last and it can take 2 years to reverse everything.
On the photo montage above, the first image is at 1 month of treatment. The middle at 4 months and the right at 7 months.
On the bottom pictures, the left shows the frontal area at 1 month, the right after only 5 months of treatment. The hair gets thicker and appears darker. There is definitely less white hair.

PART 4

SOME ANTI-AGEING PROGRAMMES

Source: C.DALLE - Le guide pratique de la médecine anti âge

My programme:

Thyroidal hormones Euthryal and Levothyrox
Hyrdocortisone 10mg in the morning
DHEA 25mg
Pregnenolone 50mg
Testosterone enanthate 80mg per week
Coenzyme q10 (Ubiquinol) 100mg
Melatonin MZS from Dr. Pierpaoli 3mg at bedtime
Niacinamide 1g
Fatty acid EPA/DHA 1g
Finasteride 1.25mg (alopecia)
Complex vitamin Maxi Hair Plus
Lysine 1g
Potassium citrate 200mg
Taurine 1g
Magnesium 300mg
Vitamin D (Zyma D) 6000 UI
Nettle leaf 400mg
Perilla Frutescens leaves in infusion

Occasionally: secretagogue of type MK677 or Glycine at bedtime, vitamin E 400mg, progesterone cream (prostate protection), Astaxanthine

Sport: weight training 2-3 times per week

Dr Thierry Hertoghe (Belgique):

Liposome testosterone gel 10%, 1 dose
Pregnenolone 50mg
Melatonin 0.5mg sublingual
Armour Thyroid 90mg
Hydrocortisone 30mg
9-alpha-fludrocortisone 100mg
DHEA 40mg
Finasteride 2.5mg (alopecia)
Progesterone 100mg
Growth hormone 0.01 UI
Vitamin E 400mg
Coenzyme Q10 100mg
Carnitine 4g
Multivitamin complex
Omega 3 EPA/DHA

Daily physical exercise
Relaxation

Dr Claude Chauchard (France)

DHEA 25mg
Vitamin E 400 UI
Potassium 600mg
Advodart (against alopecia)
Alpha-Lipoic acid/Biotine 250mg

Beta-carotene 25000 UI
Zeaxanthine
Omega 3 EPA/DHA
Lycopene 15mg
Acetyl-L carnitine 600mg
N-Acetylcysteine 600mg
L glutamine 500mg
Digestive enzymes 800mg

FINAL WORDS.

So, there you have it! We come to the end of this guide on anti-aging, also known as Functional and Nutritional Medicine.

I hope that reading this book has encouraged you to take control of your own health. Most importantly because it belongs to you and on the other hand, you possess the one key to achieve it that your doctor doesn't: time.

Do your own research, talk about it with those around you, it's essential in this world of nutrition that is constantly evolving.

With this book you have invaluable information to help you improve your help. If you still have questions however, do not hesitate to contact me by email at the following address: darkbloom987@gmail.com and I will try my best to respond to them. Similarly, do not forget to leave a review on Amazon (a positive one is favorable !), it will help my book to receive more visibility.

Do not forget: in medicine, as in other areas, there is no established truth and this applies to everyone. We are all perpetual "seekers" in search of what Hippocrates called **"the cause of causes"**.

BIBLIOGRAPHY

1 Coles LD[1], Tuite PJ[2], Öz G[3], Mishra UR[1], Kartha RV[1], Sullivan KM[1], Cloyd JC[1], Terpstra M[3].1- Gerontol A Biol Sci Med Sci. 2012 Jun;67(6):573-83. doi: 10.1093/gerona/glr208. Epub 2011 Dec 9.

Advanced glycation end-products as markers of aging and longevity in the long-lived Ansell's mole-rat (Fukomys anselli).

Dammann P[1], Sell DR, Begall S, Strauch C, Monnier VM.

2- Biosci Rep. 1999 Dec;19(6):581-7.

Carnosine, the protective, anti-aging peptide.

Boldyrev AA[1], Gallant SC, Sukhich GT.

3- J Clin Pharmacol. 2018 Feb;58(2):158-167. doi: 10.1002/jcph.1008. Epub 2017 Sep 22.

Repeated-Dose Oral N-Acetylcysteine in Parkinson's Disease: Pharmacokinetics and Effect on Brain Glutathione and Oxidative Stress.

Coles LD[1], Tuite PJ[2], Öz G[3], Mishra UR[1], Kartha RV[1], Sullivan KM[1], Cloyd JC[1], Terpstra M[3].

4- Miller ER, Pastor-Barriuso R, Dalal D, Riemersma RA, Appel LJ, Guallar E. Meta-analysis: **high-dosage vitamin E supplementation may increase all-cause mortality.** *Ann Intern Med. 2005 Jan 4;142(1):37-46.*

5- *Semin Immunol.* 2015 May;27(3):184-93. doi: 10.1016/j.smim.2015.03.013. Epub 2015 Apr 10.
Atherosclerosis - A matter of unresolved inflammation.
Viola J[1], Soehnlein O[2].

6- *ARTE : **Cholestérol : le grand bluff***

7- ***Cholestérol : mensonges et propagande***, Michel de Lorgeril, MD Ed. Thierry Souccar

8- *Lettre du Dr Thierry Hertoghe:* **Préserver ses télomères**.

9- *Michel de Lorgeril, 2018:* **L'espérance de vie régresse dans toute l'Europe, comme aux USA**. *Blog michel.delorgeril.info*

10- *Pr Philippe Even, Pr Bernard Debré, Ed. Cherche midi, 2012*: **Guide des 4000 médicaments utiles, inutiles ou dangereux.**

11- *Source : wikipédia :* **sarcopénie ou syndrome gériatrique**.

12- *"**Lait : mensonges et propagande**" Thierry Souccar.*

13- *Walter Pierpaoli, MD, PhD* **"The melatonine miracle"**.

14- *Venesson J.* **"Gluten: comment le blé moderne nous intoxique"**.

15- **Metformin reduces all-cause mortality and diseases of ageing independent of its effect on diabetes control: A systematic review and meta-analysis.**
Campbell JM, Bellman SM, Stephenson MD, Lisy K.
Ageing Res Rev. 2017 Nov;40:31-44. doi: 10.1016/j.arr.2017.08.003. Epub 2017 Aug 10.

16- CA Cancer J Clin. 2016 Mar-Apr;66(2):91-2. doi: 10.3322/caac.21299. Epub 2016 Jan 11.
Nicotinamide found to reduce the rate of nonmelanoma skin cancers in high-risk patients.
Barton MK.
*17- Benoit Claeys, MD - **En finir avec l'hypothyroïdie**, 2015 Ed. Thierry Souccar*

*18- Wentz Isabella PharmaD - **Hashimoto's hypothyroiditis. Lifestyle interventions for finding and treating the root cause.***

*19- Santé Nature Innovation 31/10/2014 - **Comment va votre thyroïde ?***

*20- Reddy D.S., Kulkarni S.K., **Neurosteroid coadministration prevents development of tolerance and augments recovery from benzodiazepine withdrawal anxiety and hyperactivity in mice.** Methods Find Exp Clin Pharmacol. 1997 Jul-Aug;19(6):395-405*

*21- Reddy D.S., Kulkarni S.K., **Differential anxiolytic effects of neurosteroids in the mirrored chamber behavior test in mice.** Brain Res.*
1997 Mar 28;752(1-2):61-71.

*22- Morley J.E., Kaiser F., Raum W.J., Perry H.M. 3rd, Flood J.F., Jensen J., Silver A.J., Roberts E., **Potentially predictive and manipulable blood serum correlates of aging in the healthy human male: progressive decreases in bioavailable testosterone, dehydroepiandrosterone sulfate, and the ratio of insulin-like growth factor 1 to growth hormone.** Proc Natl Acad Sci USA. 1997 Jul 8;94(14):7537-42.*

23- Freeman H., Pincus G., Bachrach S., Johnson C.W., McCabe G.E., MacGilpin H.H. Jr., **Oral steroid medication in rheumatoid arthritis.**
J Clin Endocrinol Metab. 1950 Dec;10(12):1523-32.

24- Mayo W., Le Moal M., Abrous D.N., **Pregnenolone sulfate and aging of cognitive functions: behavioral, neurochemical, and morphological investigations.** *Horm Behav. 2001 Sep;40(2):215-7.*

*25- John R. Lee, MD. "***Hormone balance for men : what your doctor may not tell you about prostate health and natural hormone supplementation.***"*

*26- E.Louis "***Jeunesse illimitée***" Editions Full Wellness.*

27- https://www.express.co.uk/news/uk/558249/statins-expert-heart-drug-rory-collins

*28- Dr Ronald Klatz "***Growing young with HGH***" HarperCollins Publishers*

29 - Djurhuus CB, Gravholt CH, Nielsen S, Mengel A, Christiansen JS, Schmitz OE, Møller N. **Effects of cortisol on lipolysis and regional interstitial glycerol levels in humans.** *Am J Physiol Endocrinol Metab. 2002 Jul;283(1):E172-7.*

30- Shuto M, Higuchi K, Sugiyama C, Yoneyama M, Kuramoto N, Nagashima R, Kawada K, Ogita K. **Endogenous and exogenous glucocorticoids prevent trimethyltin from causing neuronal degeneration of the mouse brain in vivo: involvement of oxidative stress pathways.** *J Pharmacol Sci. 2009 Aug;110(4):424-36.*

31- Gavan N, Maibach H. **Effect of topical corticosteroids on the activity of superoxide dismutase in human skin in vitro.** *Skin*

Pharmacol. 1997;10(5-6):309-13.

*32- Dandona P, Thusu K, Hafeez R, Abdel-Rahman E, Chaudhuri A. **Effect of hydrocortisone on oxygen free radical generation by mononuclear cells.** Metabolism. 1998 Jul;47(7):788-91.*

*33- Lettre du Dr Thierry Hertoghe N°18 "**Perte de cheveux".***

*34- Schnohr P, Nyboe J, Lange P, Jensen G. **Longevity and gray hair, baldness, facial wrinkles, and arcus senilis in 13,000 men and women: the Copenhagen City Heart Study.** J Gerontol A Biol Sci Med Sci. 1998 Sep;53(5):M347-50. (2.5 x more mortality from ischemic heart disease, and 72% more risk of disease in men with severe baldness (frontal or vertex).*

*35- Trevisan M, Farinaro E, Krogh V, Jossa F, Giumetti D, Fusco G, Panico S, Mellone C, Frascatore S, Scottoni A, et al. **Baldness and coronary heart disease risk factors**. J Clin Epidemiol. 1993 Oct;46(10):1213-8. (Participants with fronto-occipital baldness (male-type baldness) have higher cholesterol and BP).*

*36- **Somebody's Method to regrow your hair**: BOOK IS ABOUT MY HAIR LOSS TREATMENT AND HOW I WAS ABLE TO REGROW MY HAIR IN LESS THAN 7 MONTHS (English Edition) Format Kindle, Amazon download.*

NOTES

www.ingramcontent.com/pod-product-compliance
Lightning Source LLC
Chambersburg PA
CBHW051750250726
48659CB00001B/337